HANDBOOK OF FLUID, ELECTROLYTE, AND ACID-BASED IMBALANCES

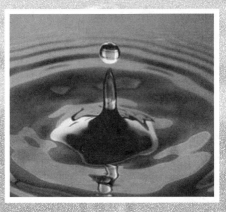

Joyce LeFever Kee, RN, MS
Associate Professor Emerita
College of Health and Nursing Science
University of Delaware
Newark, Delaware

Betty J. Paulanka, RN, EdD
Dean and Professor
College of Health and Nursing Science
University of Delaware
Newark, Delaware

Delmar Publishers

an International Thomson Publishing company I(T)P®

Albany • Bonn • Boston • Cincinnati • Detroit • London • Madrid
Melbourne • Mexico City • New York • Pacific Grove • Paris • San Francisco
Singapore • Tokyo • Toronto • Washington

P9-DFT-258

Notice to the Reader

Publisher does not warrant or guarantee any of the products described herein or perform any independent analysis in connection with any of the product information contained herein. Publisher does not assume, and expressly disclaims, any obligation to obtain and include information other than that provided to it by the manufacturer.

The reader is expressly warned to consider and adopt all safety precautions that might be indicated by the activities herein and to avoid all potential hazards. By following the instructions contained herein, the reader willingly assumes all risks in connection with such instructions. The publisher makes no representation or warranties of any kind, including but not limited to, the warranties of fitness for particular purpose or merchantability, nor are any such representations implied with respect to the material set forth herein, and the publisher takes no responsibility with respect to such material. The publisher shall not be liable for any special, consequential, or exemplary damages resulting, in whole or part, from the readers' use of, or reliance upon, this material.

Cover Design: Scott Keidong's Image Enterprises

Delmar Staff

Publisher: William Brottmiller
Acquisitions Editor: Cathy L. Esperti
Developmental Editor: Patricia A. Gaworecki
Project Editor: Patricia Gillivan

Production Coordinator: Barbara A. Bullock
Art and Design Coordinator: Timothy J. Conners
Editorial Assistant: Darcy M. Scelsi

Copyright © 2000
By Delmar Publishers Inc.

an International Thomson Publishing company I(T)P

The ITP logo is a trademark under license.
Printed in Canada

For more information, contact:

Delmar Publishers
3 Columbia Circle, Box 15015
Albany, New York 12212-5015
International Thomson Publishing Europe
Berkshire House 168-173
High Holborn
London, WC1V7AA
England
Thomas Nelson Australia
102 Dodds Street
South Melbourne, 3205
Victoria, Australia
Nelson Canada
1120 Birchmount Road
Scarborough, Ontario
Canada, MIK 5G4

International Thomson Editores
Campos Eliseos 385, Piso 7
Col Polanco
11560 Mexico D F Mexico
International Thomson Publishing GmbH
Königswinterer Strasse 418
53227 Bonn
Germany
International Thomson Publishing Asia
60 Albert Street
#15-01 Albert Complex
Singapore 189969
International Thomson Publishing—Japan
Hirakawa-cho Kyowa Building, 3F
2-2-1 Hirakawa-cho
Chiyoda-ku, Tokyo 102
Japan

All rights reserved. No part of this work covered by the copyright hereon may be reproduced or used in any form or by any means—graphic, electronic, or mechanical, including photocopying, recording, taping, or information storage and retrieval systems—without the written permission of the publisher.

1 2 3 4 5 6 7 8 9 10 XXX 05 04 03 02 01 00 99

Library of Congress Cataloging-in-Publication Data
Handbook of fluid, electrolyte, and acid-base imbalances /
 Joyce LeFever Kee, Betty J. Paulanka.
     p.   cm.
     Includes bibliographical references and index.
     ISBN 0-7668-0333-3
     1. Body fluid disorders—Handbooks, manuals, etc. 2. Acid-base imbalances—Handbooks, manuals, etc. 3. Water-electrolyte imbalances—Handbooks, manuals, etc. I. Kee, Joyce LeFever.
 II. Paulanka, Betty J.
     [DNLM: 1. Water-Electrolyte Imbalance handbooks.   2. Acid-Base Imbalance handbooks.   3. Body Fluids handbooks.   WD 200.1 H236 2000]
RC630.H36 2000
616.3'992—dc21
DNLM/DLC
for Library of Congress

98-52766
CIP

Dedication

To

My Children—Eric, Katherine, and Wanda

Joyce LeFever Kee

To

My Children—Christie and Elaine

Betty J. Paulanka

Contents

Preface

The *Handbook of Fluid, Electrolyte, and Acid-Base Imbalances* is developed from a parent text, *Fluids and Electrolytes with Clinical Applications: A Programmed Approach,* 6E by Joyce LeFever Kee and Betty J. Paulanka, and is designed to be used in the clinical setting, both in conjunction with the parent text and as a stand-alone product. With a clear comprehensive approach, this quick reference pocket guide of basic principles of fluid, electrolyte, and acid-based balances, imbalances, and related disorders is a must-have for all who work in the field! The convenient handbook size enables readers to keep it handy for quick access to over 200 diagrams and tables containing valuable information. A developmental approach is used to provide examples across the life span that illustrate common health problems associated with imbalances. Nursing assessments, diagnoses, interventions, and rationales are in a tabular format for quick retrieval and ease of comprehension. All the important information readers need is right at their fingertips!

Organization

Handbook of Fluid, Electrolyte, and Acid-Base Imbalances comprises 19 chapters organized into 5 units:

Unit I lays the foundation for influence of fluids on the body. It covers fluid imbalances related to extracellular fluid volume deficit, excess, and fluid shift, and intracellular fluid volume excess.

Unit II builds upon this material and discusses six electrolyte imbalances—potassium, sodium, chloride, calcium, magnesium, phosphorus.

Unit III provides a quick guide to determine the type of acid-base imbalances.

Unit IV covers intravenous therapy. The chapters on intravenous fluid therapy and total parenteral nutrition (TPN) include: calculation, monitoring IV fluids, and complications that may occur. With this strong foundation, the learner can then move on to the more complex issues found in the next unit.

Unit V on Fluid, Electrolyte, and Acid-Base Imbalances in Clinical Situations outlines the causes of fluid, electrolyte, and acid-base imbalances in a brief reference style format. Chapters related to acute disorders (trauma and shock), gastrointestinal surgical interventions and chronic diseases such as heart failure, diabetic ketoacidosis, and chronic obstructive pulmonary disease are included. Also addressed are the fluid problems of infants and children, and older adults.

Appendix contains 7 appendices. These act as invaluable reference tools for the user. Contained within the appendix are clinical pathways for CHF and children with fluid and electrolyte imbalances; common laboratory tests and values for adults and children; foods rich in potassium, sodium, calcium, magnesium, chloride, and phosphorus; and so much more.

Symbols

Throughout the handbook the following symbols are used: ↑ (increased), ↓ (decreased), > (greater than), < (less than). A dagger (†) in tables indicates the most common signs and symptoms.

The content in this book is geared for nurses (student, licensed, practitioner), laboratory personnel, technicians, and all health professionals wanting to learn more about fluid, electrolyte, and acid-base imbalances that influence the health status of their clients.

Joyce L. Kee, RN, MS
Betty J. Paulanka, RN, EdD, Dean

Acknowledgments

We wish to extend our deepest appreciation to Ellen Boyda, Linda Laskowski-Jones, Larry Purnell, Gail Wade, and Olga Ward for their contributions and assistance; to S. Francis Hospital, Wilmington, Delaware, for the use of their Clinical Pathways for Clients with Congestive Heart Failure, and to Christiana Care, Visiting Nurse Association, Wilmington, Delaware, for the use of their Clinical Pathways for the Newborn with Hyperbilirubinemia.

We especially wish to thank Don Passidomo, Head Librarian at the V.A. Medical Center, Wilmington, Delaware, for his valuable assistance and service and for the literature search on fluids and electrolytes.

We also offer our thanks to our editors Cathy L. Esperti and Patricia Gaworecki at Delmar Publishers for their helpful suggestions and assistance.

Joyce LeFever Kee, RN, MS
Betty J. Paulanka, RN, EdD

Contributors and Consultants

Ellen B. Boyda, RN, MS, CRNP
Family Nurse Practitioner
Pulmonary Clinical Nurse Specialist
Independent Practice
Boothwyn, PA
Metabolic Acidosis and Alkalosis
Respiratory Acidosis and Alkalosis

Linda Laskowski-Jones, RN, MS, CS, CCRN
Trauma Clinical Specialist
Trauma Service
Christiana Care Health Systems
Wilmington, Delaware
Trauma and Shock

Larry Purnell, RN, PhD
Associate Professor
College of Health and Nursing Sciences
University of Delaware
Newark, Delaware
Gastrointestinal Surgical Interventions

Gail H. Wade, RN, MS
Assistant Professor
College of Health and Nursing Sciences
University of Delaware
Newark, Delaware
Fluid Problems of Infants and Children

Olga Ward, RN
Parenteral Therapist
Christiana Care Health System
Wilmington, Delaware
Intravenous Therapy

Reviewers

Sandra Cawley Baird, EdD, RN, CNS
Director, Professor
School of Nursing
University of Northern Colorado

Carol Della Ratta, RN, MS, CCRN
Clinical Assistant Professor
State University of New York at Stony Brook

Kathie Doyle, RN, MS
Adjunct Nursing Faculty
Maria College *and* Regents College
Albany, New York

▶ INTRODUCTION

The human body is a complex machine that contains hundreds of bones and the most sophisticated interaction of systems of any structure on earth. Yet, the substance that is basic to the very existence of the body is the simplest substance known, WATER. In fact, it makes up almost two-thirds of an adult's body weight.

Body water represents about 60% of the total body weight in the average adult, 54% of an older adult, 77% of a newborn infant, and 97% of the early human embryo. Figure U1-1 demonstrates the percentage of body water concentration across the life span. Many persons think the extra water in infants acts as a protective mechanism. Since infants have larger body surface in relation to their weight, extra water acts as a cushion against injury. Body fat is essentially free of water. An obese person has less body water than a thin person. The leaner the individual, the greater the proportion of water in total body weight.

▶ BODY COMPARTMENTS

Body water is distributed among three body compartments: intracellular (within the cells), intravascular (within the blood vessels), and interstitial (within the tissue spaces). Because fluids in the blood vessels and tissue spaces are outside the cells, they are referred to as extracellular fluid. Table U1-1 gives the proportion of intracellular and extracellular fluid in the body.

▶ FUNCTIONS OF BODY WATER

Without water, the body is unable to maintain life. Five functions of water that the body needs to maintain a healthy state are stated in Table U1-2.

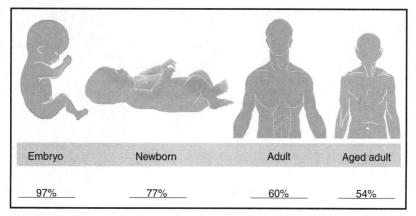

Embryo	Newborn	Adult	Aged adult
97%	77%	60%	54%

Figure U1-1 Percentages of Body Fluid per Body Weight

Table U1-1

Percentage of Body Fluids in Body Fluid Compartments

Intracellular fluid (ICF) compartment ($\frac{2}{3}$)		40%
Extracellular fluid (ECF) compartment ($\frac{1}{3}$)		20%
Interstitial fluid	15%	
Intravascular fluid	5%	
	Total	60%

Table U1-2

Functions of Body Water

- Transportation of nutrients, electrolytes, and oxygen to the cells
- Excretion of waste products
- Regulation of body temperature
- Lubrication of joints and membranes
- Medium for food digestion

When body water is insufficient and the kidneys are functioning normally, urine volume diminishes and the individual becomes thirsty. Therefore, the person drinks more water to correct the fluid deficit. When there is an excessive amount of water intake, the urine output increases proportionately.

Table U1-3

Daily Body Fluid Intake and Losses

Fluid Intake		Fluid Losses	
Liquid	1000–1200 mL	Urine	1200–1400 mL
Food	800–1000 mL	Feces	100 mL
Oxidation	200–300 mL	Lungs	400–500 mL
		Skin	300–500 mL
Total	2000–2500 mL		2000–2500 mL

Sources of fluid intake include liquids, foods, and products of the oxidation of food process. The average intake and output of fluid per day is 2000–2500 mL. Body fluids are lost daily through the urine, feces, lungs, and skin. Body water loss through the skin, which is not measurable, is called *insensible perspiration*. Appropriately 300–500 mL of fluid is lost daily through processes such as sweat gland activity. Table U1-3 lists the daily fluid intake and losses. Definitions related to fluid functions and movement are presented in the accompanying box.

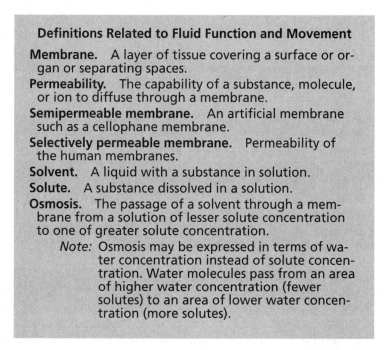

Definitions Related to Fluid Function and Movement

Membrane. A layer of tissue covering a surface or organ or separating spaces.

Permeability. The capability of a substance, molecule, or ion to diffuse through a membrane.

Semipermeable membrane. An artificial membrane such as a cellophane membrane.

Selectively permeable membrane. Permeability of the human membranes.

Solvent. A liquid with a substance in solution.

Solute. A substance dissolved in a solution.

Osmosis. The passage of a solvent through a membrane from a solution of lesser solute concentration to one of greater solute concentration.

Note: Osmosis may be expressed in terms of water concentration instead of solute concentration. Water molecules pass from an area of higher water concentration (fewer solutes) to an area of lower water concentration (more solutes).

Diffusion. The movement of molecules such as gas from an area of higher concentration to an area of lesser concentration. Large molecules move less rapidly than small molecules.

Osmol. A unit of osmotic pressure. The osmotic effects are expressed in terms of osmolality. A **milliosmol (mOsm)** is 1/1000th of an osmol and determines the osmotic activity.

Osmolality. Osmotic pull exerted by all particles per unit of water, expressed as osmols or milliosmols per kilogram of water.

Osmolarity. Osmotic pull exerted by all particles per unit of solution, expressed as osmols or milliosmols per liter of solution.

Ion. A particle carrying a positive or negative charge.

Plasma. Blood minus the blood cells (composed mainly of water).

Serum. Plasma minus fibrogen (obtained after coagulation of blood).

Tonicity. The effect of fluid on cellular volume.

▶ FLUID PRESSURES (STARLING'S LAW)

Extracellular fluid (ECF) shifts between the intravascular space (blood vessels) and the interstitial space (tissues) to maintain a fluid balance within the ECF compartment. There are four measurable pressures that determine the flow of fluid between the intravascular and interstitial spaces. These are the colloid osmotic (oncotic) pressures and the hydrostatic pressures that occur in both the vessels and the tissue spaces. The colloid osmotic pressure and the hydrostatic pressure of the blood and tissues influence the movement of fluid through the capillary membrane. Fluid exchange occurs only across the walls of capillaries and not across the walls of arterioles or venules. Therefore, fluid moves into the interstitial space at the arteriolar end of the capillary and out of the interstitial space into the capillary at the venular end of the capillary.

Fluid flows only when there is a difference in pressure at the two ends of the system. The difference in pressure between two points is known as the pressure gradient. If the pressure at one end is 32 mm Hg and at the other end is 26 mm Hg, the pressure gradient is 6 mm Hg. The plasma in the capillaries has hydrostatic pressure and colloid osmotic pressure. The tissue fluids have hydrostatic pressure and colloid osmotic pressure. The difference of pressure between the plasma colloid osmotic pressure and the tissue colloid osmotic pressure is known as the colloid osmotic pressure gradient; likewise, the difference of pressure between the plasma hy-

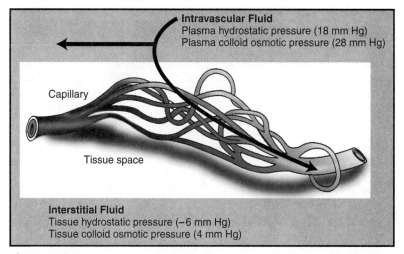

Figure U1-2 Pressures in the Intravascular and Interstitial Fluid

drostatic pressure and the tissue hydrostatic pressure is known as the hydrostatic pressure gradient. Figure U1-2 describes the fluid flow based upon the pressures in the intravascular and interstitial spaces.

Because the plasma hydrostatic pressure (18 mm Hg) in the arteriolar end of the capillary is higher than the tissue hydrostatic pressure (−6 mm Hg) in the tissue spaces, fluid moves out of the capillary and into the tissue spaces. The plasma colloid osmotic pressure (28 mm Hg) in the venular end of the capillary is higher than the tissue colloid osmotic pressure (4 mm Hg) in the tissue spaces, causing fluids to move from the tissue spaces into the capillary. Without the colloid osmotic forces, fluid is lost from circulation and remains in the tissues, causing swelling or edema.

▶ REGULATORS OF FLUID BALANCE

Thirst, electrolytes, protein and albumin, hormones, enzymes, lymphatics, skin, and kidneys are major regulators that maintain body fluid balance. Thirst alerts the person that there is a fluid loss; thus, thirst stimulates the person to increase his or her oral intake. The thirst mechanism in the medulla may not respond effectively to a fluid deficit in the older adult or the very young child; therefore, these groups of individuals are prone to lose fluid and become easily dehydrated. Table U1-4 lists the various regulators of fluid balance. The body compensates for fluid changes.

If a person is febrile or there is an increase in humidity, diaphoresis may occur. This causes a fluid loss. The amount of fluid loss from the skin in this situation may be greater than 500 mL for the day. Deep and rapid breathing or hyperventilation can also increase fluid loss through the lungs in an amount greater than 500 mL.

Table U1-4

Regulators of Fluid Balance

Regulators	Actions
Thirst	An indicator of fluid need.
Electrolytes and Nonelectrolytes	
Sodium	Sodium promotes water retention. With a water deficit, less sodium is excreted via kidneys; thus, more water is retained.
Protein, albumin	Protein and albumin promote body fluid retention. These nondiffusible substances increase the colloid osmotic (oncotic) pressure in favor of fluid retention.
Hormones and Enzymes	
Antidiuretic hormone (ADH)	ADH is produced by the hypothalamus and stored in the posterior pituitary gland (neurohypophysis). ADH is secreted when there is an ECF volume deficit or an increased osmolality (increased solutes). ADH promotes water reabsorption from the distal tubules of the kidneys.
Aldosterone	Aldosterone is secreted from the adrenal cortex. It promotes sodium, chloride, and water reabsorption from the renal tubules.
Renin	Decreased renal blood flow increases the release of renin, an enzyme, from the juxtaglomerular cells of the kidneys. Renin promotes peripheral vasoconstriction and the release of aldosterone (sodium and water retention).
Body Tissues and Organs	
Lymphatics	Plasma protein that shifts to the tissue spaces cannot be reabsorbed into the blood vessels. Thus, the lymphatic system promotes the return of water and protein from the interstitial spaces to the vascular spaces.
Skin	Skin excretes approximately 300–500 mL of water daily through normal perspiration.
Lungs	Lungs excrete approximately 400–500 mL of water daily through normal breathing.
Kidneys	The kidneys excrete 1000–1500 mL of body water daily. The amount of water excretion may vary according to the balance between fluid intake and fluid loss.

▶ OSMOLALITY

Osmolality (serum) is determined by the number of dissolved particles, mainly sodium, urea, and glucose, per kilogram of water. Sodium is the largest contributor of particles to osmolality. The normal serum osmolality range is 280–295 mOsm/kg (milliosmols per kilogram); serum osmolality values in this range are considered iso-osmolar since the serum concentration is similar to plasma. If the serum osmolality is less than (<) 280 mOsm/kg, the serum concentration of fluid is hypo-osmolar, and if the serum osmolality is greater than (>) 295 mOsm/kg, the serum concentration is hyperosmolar. The serum osmolality is "roughly" estimated by doubling the serum sodium level. For example, if the serum sodium is 142 mEq/L, the serum osmolality is 284 mOsm/kg. Doubling the serum sodium level provides a "rough estimate" of the serum osmolality. Another formula that is more accurate in determining the serum osmolality is displayed in the accompanying box. If the client's serum sodium is 140 mEq/L, blood urea nitrogen (BUN) is 12 mg/dL, and serum glucose is 99 mg/dL, the serum osmolality for this client is 289.5 mOsm/kg; the serum concentration is iso-osmolar or iso-osmolality.

Formula for Calculating Serum Osmolality

$$2 \times \text{serum sodium} + \frac{BUN}{3} + \frac{glucose}{18} = \text{serum osmolality}$$

Rough Estimation of Serum Osmolality

$$2 \times \text{serum sodium} = \text{serum osmolality}$$

Use the formula in the accompanying box for clients A and B. Client A: The serum sodium is 145 mEq/L, BUN is 27 mg/dL, and the serum glucose is 120 mg/dL. Client A's serum osmolality is 305.7 or 306 mOsm/kg, which shows hyperosmolality. Client B: The serum sodium is 133 mEq/L, BUN is 9 mg/dL, and the serum glucose is 90 mg/dL. Client B's serum osmolality is 274 mOsm/kg, which shows hypo-osmolality.

The terms osmolality and tonicity have been used interchangeably; though similar, they are different. **Osmolality** is the concentration of body fluids and **tonicity** is the effect of fluid on cellular volume. Increased osmolality (hyperosmolality) can result from impermeant solutes such as sodium and permeant solutes such as urea (blood urea nitrogen). Hypertonicity results from an increase of impermeant solutes such as sodium, but *not* of permeant solutes such as urea (BUN). Hyperosmolality of body fluid occurs with an increased serum sodium and BUN levels; however, it may also cause isotonicity since the BUN does not affect tonicity. Serum osmolality is a better indicator of the concentration of solutes in body fluids than tonicity measures. Tonicity is primarily used for the concentration of intavenous solutions.

▶ OSMOLALITY OF INTRAVENOUS (IV) SOLUTION

The osmolality of an IV solution can be hypo-osmolar or hypotonic, iso-osmolar or isotonic, hyperosmolar or hypertonic. The osmolality of an IV solution is determined by the serum osmolality average, which is 290 mOsm/kg (280–295 mOsm/kg). The normal range for the osmolality of a solution is +50 mOsm or −50 mOsm of 290 mOsm, or 240–340 mOsm. Tonicity may be used to describe the concentration of IV solution because of the effect of impermeant solutes like sodium and chloride in the solution on the cellular volume. Since the solute concentration is determined by the number of osmols or milliosmols in solution, hypo-osmolar, iso-osmolar, and hyperosmolar are the suggested terms.

A liter of 5% dextrose in water (D_5W) is 250 mOsm, and a liter of 0.9% sodium chloride or normal saline is 310 mOsm; both solutions have somewhat the same osmolality as plasma. These solutions are iso-osmolar. However, in D_5W, the dextrose is metabolized quickly, causing the solution to become hypo-osmolar. The osmolality of a liter of 5% dextrose in water with 0.9% sodium chloride is 560 mOsm. This solution is hyperosmolar.

Many disease entities have some degree of fluid imbalance such as fluid loss, fluid excess, and/or fluid volume shift. The four major fluid imbalances: extracellular fluid volume deficit (ECFVD), extracellular fluid volume excess (ECFVE), extracellular fluid volume shift (ECFVS), and intracellular fluid volume excess (ICFVE) are discussed in Chapters 1, 2, 3, and 4.

Extracellular Fluid Volume Deficit (ECFVD)

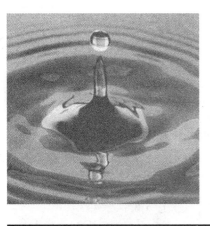

❯ INTRODUCTION

Extracellular fluid volume deficit (ECFVD) indicates a loss of body fluid from the interstitial (tissue) and/or intravascular (vascular–blood vessel) spaces. When there is a *severe* extracellular fluid loss and the serum osmolality is increased (more solutes than water), the fluid in the intracellular (cells) is greatly decreased. Hyperosmolality pulls water out of the cells to maintain homeostasis (equilibrium) of the body fluid and cellular dehydration results. If serum osmolality remains normal (loss of water and the loss of solutes is equal), intracellular fluid loss is unlikely to occur.

Dehydration means lack of water. Dehydration may occur due to extracellular fluid loss or a decreased fluid intake. An elevated serum osmolality occurs frequently with dehydration. The serum osmolality can be closely estimated using the serum sodium, BUN, and glucose values presented in Unit I.

▶ PATHOPHYSIOLOGY

A loss of the electrolyte sodium is usually accompanied by a loss of extracellular fluid. The extracellular fluid is usually decreased or moves from the ECF to the ICF (intracellular fluid) compartment. When fluid and sodium are lost in equal amounts, the type of fluid deficit that usually occurs is **iso-osmolar** (iso-osmolar fluid volume deficit). The serum osmolality remains in normal range between 280 and 295 mOsm/kg, as shown in the accompanying box. If the amount of water loss is in excess of the amount of sodium loss, the serum sodium level is increased. This type of fluid deficit is called a **hyperosmolar** fluid volume deficit. With the retention of sodium or loss of water, serum osmolality increases (>295 mOsm/kg). Hyperosmolar extracellular fluid causes intracellular dehydration because the increase in serum osmolality causes water to be drawn from the cells. With an iso-osmolar fluid volume loss, the loss of water and solute is equal. An iso-osmolar fluid volume loss is not classified as dehydration, although dehydration can occur with this type of fluid loss. Table 1-1 differentiates between iso-osmolar fluid volume deficit and hyperosmolar fluid volume deficit.

Normal serum osmolality: 280–295 mOsm/kg

Hypo-osmolality:	<280 mOsm/kg
Iso-osmolality:	280–295 mOsm/kg
Hyperosmolality:	>295 mOsm/kg

Table 1-1

Differentiation between Iso-osmolar and Hyperosmolar Fluid Volume Deficit

Situation	Iso-osmolar Fluid Volume Deficit	Hyperosmolar Fluid Volume deficit
There is a proportional loss of both body fluids and solutes	X	
The loss of body fluid is greater than the loss of solutes		X
A serum osmolality of 282 mOsm/kg occurs with ECFVD	X	
A serum osmolality of 320 mOsm/kg occurs with ECFVD		X

Compensatory mechanisms such as increased heart rate and blood pressure attempt to maintain the fluid volume necessary for vital organs to receive adequate perfusion. When more than one-third of the body fluid is lost, vascular collapse occurs and shock results.

▶ ETIOLOGY

The causes of hyperosmolar and iso-osmolar fluid volume deficits differ. Vomiting and diarrhea may cause both types of fluid volume deficits; however, in most cases, the severity of vomiting and diarrhea indicates which type of ECFVD occurs. Table 1-2 discusses the types, causes, and rationale for ECFVDs. Table 1-3 summarizes the pathophysiology and etiology related to extracellular fluid volume deficit.

▶ CLINICAL MANIFESTATIONS

The clinical manifestations (signs and symptoms) of ECFVDs are listed in Table 1-4 (see page 14). The table describes the degrees of ECF loss, percentage of body weight loss, symptoms, and body water deficit by liter for a man weighing 150 pounds.

Thirst is a symptom that occurs with mild, marked, and severe fluid loss. Lack of water intake is the main contributing cause of mild dehydration. In the elderly, the thirst mechanism in the medulla does not alert the older person that there is a water deficit. Common symptoms of marked ECF loss include decreased skin turgor, dry mucous membranes, increased pulse rate, weight loss, and decreased urine output. With marked and severe body fluid loss, the hematocrit, hemoglobin, and blood urea nitrogen (BUN) are generally increased.

During early dehydration, the serum osmolality may not show signs of significant change. As dehydration continues, fluid is lost in greater quantities from the extracellular space than from the intracellular space. This results in an ECF deficit. When dehydration is severe, the serum osmolality increases, causing water to leave the cells. This results in cellular dehydration. A severe ECF deficit can lead to an ICF deficit.

The health professional can make a quick assessment of dehydration caused by hypovolemia by checking the peripheral veins in the hand. First hold the hand above the heart level for a short time and then lower the hand below the heart level. With a normal blood volume and circulating blood flow, the peripheral veins in the hand held below the heart level should be engorged within 5–10 seconds. If the peripheral veins do not engorge in 10 seconds, this may be indicative of dehydration or low blood volume. Body weight is another important tool for assessing fluid imbalance. Two and two-tenths (2.2) pounds of body weight loss or gain is equivalent to 1 liter of water loss or gain. Of course, in order to make

Table 1-2

Causes of Extracellular Fluid Volume Deficits

Types and Causes	Rationale
Hyperosmolar Fluid Volume Deficit	
Inadequate fluid intake	A decrease in water intake results in an increase in the numbers of solutes in body fluid. The body fluid becomes hyperosmolar.
Increased solute intake (salt, sugar, protein)	An increase in solute intake increases the solute concentration in body fluid; the body fluids can become hyperosmolar with a normal or decreased fluid intake.
Severe vomiting and diarrhea	Cause a loss of body water greater than the loss of solutes such as electrolytes, resulting in hyperosmolar body fluid.
Diabetes ketoacidosis	An increase in glucose and ketone bodies can result in body fluids becoming more hyperosmolar, thus causing diuresis. The resulting fluid loss is greater than the solute loss (sugar and ketones).
Sweating	Water loss is usually greater than sodium loss.
Iso-osmolar Fluid Volume Deficit	
Vomiting and diarrhea	Usually result in fluid losses that are in proportion to electrolyte (sodium, potassium, chloride, bicarbonate) losses.
Gastrointestinal (GI) fistula or draining abscess and GI suctioning	The GI tract is rich in electrolytes. With a loss of GI secretions, fluid and electrolytes are lost in somewhat equal proportions.
Fever, environmental temperature, and profuse diaphoresis	Result in fluid and sodium losses via the skin. With profuse sweating, the sodium is usually lost in proportions equal to water losses. Depending upon the severity of the sweating and fever, symptoms of mild, moderate, or marked fluid loss may be observed.
Hemorrhage	Excess blood loss is fluid and solute loss from the vascular fluid. If hemorrhage occurs rapidly, fluid shifts to compensate for blood losses can be inadequate.
Burns	Burns cause body fluid with solutes to shift from the vascular fluid to the burned site and surrounding interstitial space (tissues). This may result in inadequate circulating fluid volume.
Ascites	Fluid and solutes (protein, electrolytes, etc.) shift to the peritoneal space, causing ascites (third-space fluid). A decrease in circulating fluid volume may result.
Intestinal obstruction	Fluid accumulates at the intestinal obstruction site (third-space fluid), thus decreasing the vascular fluid volume.

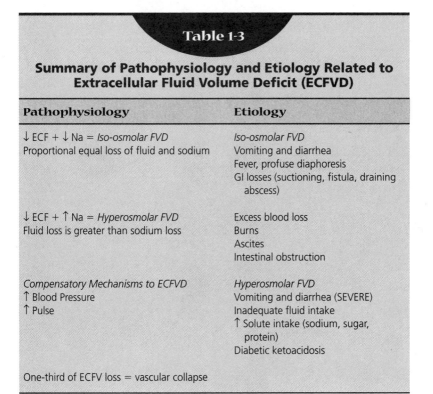

Table 1-3

Summary of Pathophysiology and Etiology Related to Extracellular Fluid Volume Deficit (ECFVD)

Pathophysiology	Etiology
↓ ECF + ↓ Na = *Iso-osmolar FVD* Proportional equal loss of fluid and sodium	*Iso-osmolar FVD* Vomiting and diarrhea Fever, profuse diaphoresis GI losses (suctioning, fistula, draining abscess)
↓ ECF + ↑ Na = *Hyperosmolar FVD* Fluid loss is greater than sodium loss	Excess blood loss Burns Ascites Intestinal obstruction
Compensatory Mechanisms to ECFVD ↑ Blood Pressure ↑ Pulse	*Hyperosmolar FVD* Vomiting and diarrhea (SEVERE) Inadequate fluid intake ↑ Solute intake (sodium, sugar, protein) Diabetic ketoacidosis
One-third of ECFV loss = vascular collapse	

an accurate assessment, the health professional needs to know the baseline body weight prior to the fluid loss.

▶ CLINICAL MANAGEMENT

In replacing body water loss, the total fluid deficit is estimated according to the percentage of body weight lost. The health care provider computes the fluid replacement for his or her client. To determine the total fluid loss, multiply the percentage of body weight loss by kilograms of body weight. If the client's weight loss is 10 pounds and his original weight was 154 pounds or 70 kg, the client has a 6% body weight loss, which totals 4.2 liters of total fluid loss. Table 1-5 gives a formula for estimating total fluid loss.

One-third of the body water deficit is from ECF (extracellular fluid) and two-thirds of the body water deficit is from ICF (intracellular fluid).

Table 1-4

Degrees of Dehydration

Degrees of Dehydration	Percentage of Body Weight Loss (%)	Symptoms	Body Water Deficit by Liter
Mild dehydration	2	1. Thirst	1–2
Marked dehydration	5	1. Marked thirst 2. Dry mucous membranes 3. Dryness and wrinkling of skin—poor skin turgor 4. Hand veins: slow filling with hand lowered 5. Temperature—low-grade elevation, e.g., 99°F (37.2°C) 6. Tachycardia (pulse greater than 100) as blood volume drops 7. Respiration >28 8. Systolic BP 10–15 mm Hg ↓ in standing position 9. Urine volume <25 mL/h 10. Specific gravity >1.030 11. Body weight loss 12. Hct ↑, Hgb ↑, BUN ↑ 13. Acid-base equilibrium toward greater acidity	3–5
Severe dehydration	8	1. Same symptoms as marked dehydration, plus: 2. Flushed skin 3. Systolic BP <60 mm Hg 4. Behavioral changes, e.g., restlessness, irritability, disorientation, and delirium	5–10
Fatal dehydration	22–30 total body water loss can prove fatal	1. Anuria 2. Coma leading to death	

Abbreviations: BP, blood pressure; Hct, hematocrit; Hgb, hemoglobin; BUN, blood urea nitrogen

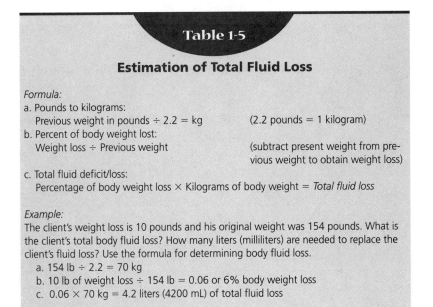

Table 1-5

Estimation of Total Fluid Loss

Formula:
a. Pounds to kilograms:
   Previous weight in pounds ÷ 2.2 = kg   (2.2 pounds = 1 kilogram)
b. Percent of body weight lost:
   Weight loss ÷ Previous weight   (subtract present weight from pre-
                                                  vious weight to obtain weight loss)
c. Total fluid deficit/loss:
   Percentage of body weight loss × Kilograms of body weight = *Total fluid loss*

Example:
The client's weight loss is 10 pounds and his original weight was 154 pounds. What is
the client's total body fluid loss? How many liters (milliliters) are needed to replace the
client's fluid loss? Use the formula for determining body fluid loss.
   a. 154 lb ÷ 2.2 = 70 kg
   b. 10 lb of weight loss ÷ 154 lb = 0.06 or 6% body weight loss
   c. 0.06 × 70 kg = 4.2 liters (4200 mL) of total fluid loss

The daily fluid loss that needs replacement is 2.5 liters or 2500 mL. During the first day the patient should receive:

$\frac{1}{3}$ × 4.2 L = 1.4 L or 1400 mL (ECF replacement)
$\frac{2}{3}$ × 4.2 L = 2.8 L or 2800 mL (ICF replacement)
2.5 L or 2500 mL to replace the current day's losses

Note: The amount for fluid replacement can vary according to the client's physical health and age. Clients with heart failure cannot receive huge fluid replacements.

Table 1-6 lists suggested solution and potassium replacement for an ECF deficit. The amount of fluid replacement might change according to the client's health status. According to Table 1-6, as potassium enters the cells, fluid flows into the cells with the potassium replacement. Cellular fluid increases and the cells become hydrated. When potassium is being administered intravenously, the client's urinary output must be closely monitored. The urine output should be at least 250 mL per 8 hours; since 80–90% of potassium is excreted by the kidneys, poor urine output results in a potassium excess.

The health care provider must also consider the electrolyte balance with different types of fluid replacement. If dextrose in water is

Table 1-6

Suggested Solution Replacement for ECF Deficit

1. Lactated Ringer's, 1500 mL, to replace ECF losses (varies according to the serum potassium and calcium levels).
2. Normal saline solution (0.9% NaCl solution), 500 mL.
3. Five percent dextrose in water (D_5W), 4700 mL, to replace the water deficit and increase urine output.
4. Potassium chloride, 40–80 mEq, may be divided into 3 liters to replace potassium loss. The serum potassium level must be closely monitored.
5. Bicarbonate as needed if an acidotic state exists.

administered without any other electrolyte content such as sodium, the dextrose is metabolized quickly, leaving only water and a resulting hypo-osmolar or hypotonic condition. An electrolyte solution such as lactated Ringer's and/or saline solution (0.9% or 0.45%) should be included as part of the replacement formula.

● Clinical Considerations: ECFVD

1. Thirst is an early symptom of ECFVD or dehydration. Encourage fluid intake.
2. The serum osmolality is one method to detect dehydration. A serum osmolality of >300 mOsm/kg indicates dehydration.
3. Decreased skin turgor, dry mucous membranes, an increased pulse rate, and a systolic blood pressure (while standing) <10–15 mm Hg of the regular blood pressure are some signs and symptoms of dehydration.
4. Urine output less than 25 mL/h or 600 mL/day should be reported. A decrease in urine output can indicate insufficient fluid intake, hypovolemia, or renal dysfunction.
5. A quick assessment of hypovolemia or dehydration can be accomplished by checking the peripheral veins in the hand. First hold the hand above the heart level for 10 seconds and then lower the hand below the heart level. The peripheral veins in the hand below the heart level become engorged within 5–10 seconds with a normal blood volume. If the peripheral veins are not engorged, hypovolemia or dehydration is present.
6. Lactated Ringer's and 5% dextrose in $\frac{1}{3}$ or $\frac{1}{2}$ normal saline are solutions that are helpful for treating ECFVD.

▶ CLIENT MANAGEMENT

Assessment

- Obtain a client history identifying factors that may cause a fluid volume deficit (ECFVD).

- Assess for signs and symptoms associated with body fluid loss or dehydration. These may include poor skin turgor, dry mucous membranes, slow filling of hand veins, a decrease in urine output, and tachycardia.

- Check vital signs. Heart compensates for fluid loss by increasing the heart rate. Check blood pressure while the client is sitting and again when standing (a fall of 10–15 mm Hg in systolic pressure can indicate marked ECFVD). A narrow pulse pressure of less than 20 mm Hg can indicate severe hypovolemia.

- Check the urine output for volume and concentration. A decrease in urine output may be due to a lack of fluid intake or excess body fluid loss.

- Assess weight gain/loss to assist in accurate fluid replacement.

- Check laboratory results of BUN and hematocrit. Elevated levels might indicate fluid loss.

Diagnoses

- *Fluid Volume Deficit Dehydration,* related to inadequate fluid intake, vomiting, diarrhea, hemorrhage, or third-space fluid loss (burns or ascites)

- *Risk for Impaired Skin Integrity,* related to a fluid deficit in body tissues

- *Altered Tissue Perfusion, renal,* related to decreased renal blood flow and poor urine output secondary to ECFVD, or hypovolemia

Interventions

- Monitor vital signs at least every 4 hours. Check the blood pressure in lying, sitting, and standing positions.

- Routinely check body weight. *Remember:* 2.2 pounds equals 1 kilogram, which is equivalent to 1 liter (1000 mL) of fluid loss.

- Monitor skin turgor, mucous membranes, lips, and tongue for dryness or improvement.

- Promote adequate fluid replacements, oral and intravenous.

- Monitor urine output. Report if urine output is below 250 mL per 8 hours.
- Provide oral hygiene several times a day.
- Monitor laboratory results such as elevated BUN and hematocrit.
- Provide comfort.
- Listen to client's concerns. Answer questions or refer the questions to appropriate health professionals.

Evaluation/Outcome

- Evaluate that the cause of extracellular fluid volume deficit (ECFVD) has been controlled or eliminated.
- Remain free of signs and symptoms of dehydration; skin turgor improved, moist mucous membranes, vital signs within normal range, and body weight increased.
- Evaluate the effects of clinical management for ECFVD; fluid deficit is lessened.
- Urine output is within normal range: 600–1400 mL/24 hours.
- Evaluate the laboratory test results; serum osmolality and electrolytes are within normal range.

Extracellular Fluid Volume Excess (ECFVE)

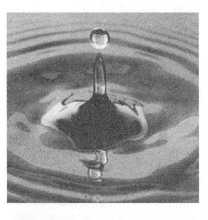

▶ INTRODUCTION

Extracellular fluid volume excess (ECFVE) is increased fluid in either the interstitial (tissues) and/or intravascular (vascular or vessel) spaces. Usually it relates to the excess fluid in tissues of the extremities (peripheral edema) or lung tissues (pulmonary edema). Terms for ECFVE are hypervolemia, overhydration, and edema. Hypervolemia and overhydration contribute to fluid excess in tissue spaces. Fluid overload is another term for overhydration and hypervolemia.

Usually edema is the abnormal retention of fluid in the interstitial spaces in the ECF compartment, but it can occur in serous cavities such as the peritoneal cavity. In edema, sodium retention is the frequent cause of the increased extracellular fluid volume. Figure 2-1 demonstrates the changes in body fluid compartments as edema occurs.

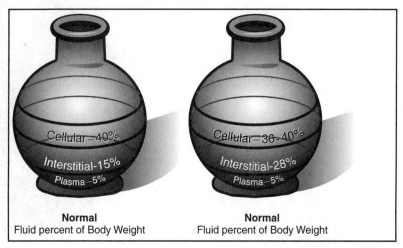

Figure 2-1 Body Fluid Compartments and Edema

▶ PATHOPHYSIOLOGY

When sodium and water are retained in the same proportion, the fluid volume excess is referred to as **iso-osmolar** fluid volume excess. Usually the serum sodium level is within the normal range. If only free water is retained, the fluid volume excess is referred to as **hypo-osmolar** fluid volume excess. The serum sodium level is decreased. When there is fluid volume excess, the fluid pressure is greater than the oncotic pressure; therefore, more fluid is pushed into the tissue spaces. Table 2-1 differentiates between iso-osmolar and hypo-osmolar fluid volume excess.

If the kidneys cannot excrete the excess intravascular fluid, fluid is frequently pushed into the tissue spaces and into the lung tissue spaces. Peripheral and/or pulmonary edema results. Fluid overload in the periphery will settle in the most dependent region: for example, feet and ankles when standing and sacrum when lying supine. When excess fluid crosses the alveolar-capillary membrane of the lungs, pulmonary edema results.

▶ ETIOLOGY

Edema is commonly associated with excess extracellular body fluid or excess fluid. Physiologic factors leading to edema may be caused by various clinical conditions, such as congestive heart failure (CHF), renal failure, cirrhosis of the liver, steroid excess, and allergic reaction. Table 2-2 lists the physiologic factors for edema, the rationale, and the clinical conditions associated with each physiologic factor.

Table 2-1

Differentiation Between Iso-osmolar and Hypo-osmolar Fluid Volume Excess

Situation	Iso-osmolar Fluid Volume Excess	Hypo-osmolar Fluid Volume Excess
There is a proportional gain of both body fluids and solutes (sodium)	X	
The gain of body fluid is greater than the gain of sodium		X
A serum osmolality of 284 mOsm/kg occurs with ECFVE	X	
A serum osmolality of 273 mOsm/kg occurs with ECFVE		X

As blood is "backed up" in the venous system, capillary pressure is increased, forcing more fluid into the tissue spaces. A decrease in plasma/serum protein results in a decrease in plasma colloid osmotic (oncotic) pressure. This causes water to move from the vessels into the tissue spaces. An increase in the capillary membrane permeability permits plasma proteins to escape from the capillaries; thus, more water moves into the interstitial spaces. The kidneys regulate the gain/loss of sodium, chloride, and water via the renin-angiotensin-aldosterone system. With inadequate blood flow to the kidney or renal dysfunction or the presence of excess aldosterone, sodium retention occurs. Sodium retention results in water retention.

Clients with limited cardiac or renal reserve frequently develop pulmonary edema. When the heart is not able to function adequately and the kidneys cannot excrete a sufficient amount of urine, the fluid backs up into the pulmonary circulatory system; fluid moves from the vessels into the lung tissues. Administering an excessive amount of intravenous fluids to a person in pulmonary edema will further worsen the edema in the lungs. Intravenous infusions should be restricted in clients with pulmonary edema.

Table 2-2

Physiologic Factors Leading to Edema

Physiologic Factors		Rationale	Clinical Conditions
Plasma hydrostatic pressure in the capillaries	↑ I n c r e a s e d	Blood dammed in the venous system can cause "back" pressure in capillaries, thus raising capillary pressure. Increased capillary pressure will force more fluid into tissue areas, thus producing edema.	1. Congestive heart failure with increased venous pressure. 2. Kidney failure resulting in sodium and water retention. 3. Venous obstruction leading to varicose veins. 4. Pressure on veins because of swelling, constricting bandages, casts, tumor, pregnancy.
Plasma colloid osmotic pressure	↓ D e c r e a s e d	Decreased plasma colloid osmotic pressure results from diminished plasma protein concentration. Decreased protein content may cause water to flow from plasma into tissue spaces, thus causing edema.	1. Malnutrition due to lack of protein in diet. 2. Chronic diarrhea resulting in loss of protein. 3. Burns leading to loss of fluid containing protein through denuded skin. 4. Kidney disease, particularly nephrosis. 5. Cirrhosis of liver resulting in decreased production of plasma protein. 6. Loss of plasma proteins through urine.
Capillary permeability	↑ I n c r e a s e d	Increased permeability of capillary membrane will allow plasma proteins to leak out of capillaries into interstitial space more rapidly than lymphatics can return them to circulation. Increased capillary permeability is predisposing factor to edema.	1. Bacterial inflammation causes increased porosity. 2. Allergic reactions. 3. Burns causing damage to capillaries. 4. Acute kidney disease, e.g., nephritis.

continues on the following page

Table 2-2

(Continued)

Physiologic Factors	Rationale	Clinical Conditions
Sodium retention	↑ Increased Kidneys regulate level of sodium ions in extracellular fluid. Kidney function will depend on adequate blood flow. Inadequate blood flow, presence of excess aldosterone or glucocorticosteroids, and diseased kidneys are predisposing factors to edema since they cause sodium, chloride and water retention.	1. Congestive heart failure causing inadequate circulation of blood. 2. Renal failure—inadequate circulation of blood through kidneys. 3. Increased production of adrenal cortical hormones—aldosterone, cortisone, and hydrocortisone—will cause retention of sodium. 4. Cirrhosis of liver. Diseased liver cannot destroy excess production of aldosterone. 5. Trauma resulting from fractures, burns, and surgery.
Lymphatic drainage	↓ Decreased Blockage of lymphatics will prevent return of proteins to circulation. Obstructed lymph flow is said to be high in protein content. With inadequate return of proteins to circulation, plasma colloid osmotic pressure will be decreased, thus causing edema.	1. Lymphatic obstruction, e.g., cancer of lymphatic system. 2. Surgical removal of lymph nodes. 3. Elephantiasis, which is parasitic invasion of lymph channels, resulting in fibrous tissue growing in nodes, obstructing lymph flow. 4. Obesity because of inadequate supporting structures for lymphatics in lower extremities. Muscles are considered the supporting structures.

▶ CLINICAL MANIFESTATIONS

There are numerous clinical manifestations (signs and symptoms) of ECFVE that relate to pulmonary edema and peripheral edema. When the fluid volume excess (hypervolemia or overhydration) causes a back-up of fluid that seeps into the lung tissue, pulmonary edema results. An early symptom of pulmonary edema is a constant, irritated cough. Table 2-3 lists the clinical signs and symptoms of ECFVE related to pulmonary and peripheral edema. Laboratory test results influenced by ECFVE are included. The rationale for each sign or symptom is given.

A quick assessment for hypervolemia, or overhydration, can be done by checking the peripheral veins in the hand. Instruct the client to hold a hand above the heart level. If the peripheral veins of the hand remain engorged after 10 seconds, this can be an indication of hypervolemia. When the jugular vein remains engorged after a person is in semi-Fowler's position, the cause is most likely hypervolemia. Lungs should be checked for the presence of moist rales. Cyanosis is a late symptom of pulmonary edema.

Gravity has an effect on the distribution of fluid in the edematous person. In a lying position, there is more equal distribution of edema, whereas in an upright position the edema is more prevalent in the lower extremities. This is called *dependent edema.* Dependent edema should not be present after the client has been in a prone or supine position for the night. If edema is present in the morning, it is most likely due to cardiac, renal, or liver disease and can be called *nondependent edema.* Edema that does not respond to diuretics is called *refractory edema.*

▶ CLINICAL MANAGEMENT

Normally, water alone does not cause or increase edema. Salt and water intake increases fluid retention and can cause edema. The three D's—diuretics, digoxin, and diet (low sodium)—are frequently prescribed for the clinical management of clients with ECFVE and with congestive heart failure (CHF). Table 2-4 presents the basic management with rationale for correcting edema.

● Clinical Considerations: ECFVE

1. ECFVE, overhydration or hypervolemia, usually relates to excess fluid in tissues of the extremities (peripheral edema) or lungs (pulmonary edema).
2. Body water retention (edema) usually results from sodium retention. If only free water is retained, the excess is referred to as hypoosmolar (hypotonic) fluid volume excess.

Table 2-3

Clinical Manifestations of ECFVE— Hypervolemia, Overhydration, Edema

Signs and Symptoms	Rationale
Pulmonary Edema	
Constant, irritated cough	An irritated cough is frequently the first clinical symptom of hypervolemia. It is caused by fluid "backed up" into the lungs (fluid is in the alveoli).
Dyspnea (difficulty in breathing)	Breathing is labored and difficult due to fluid congestion in lungs.
Neck vein engorgement	Jugular vein remains engorged when the patient is in semi-Fowler's or sitting position.
Sublingual vein engorgement	Engorged veins under the tongue may indicate hypervolemia.
Hand vein engorgement	Peripheral veins in the hand remain engorged with hand elevated above heart level for 10 seconds.
Moist rales in lung	Lungs are congested with fluid. Moist rales in lung can be heard with the stethoscope.
Bounding pulse	A full, bounding pulse may be present with hypervolemia. The pulse rate may increase.
Cyanosis	Can be a late symptom of pulmonary edema as a result of impaired gas exchange caused by fluid in the alveolar space.
Peripheral Edema	
Pitting edema in extremities	Peripheral edema present in the morning may result from inadequate heart, liver, or kidney function. A positive test of pitting edema is a finger indentation on the edematous area.
Tight, smooth, shiny skin over edematous area	Excess fluid in the peripheral tissues may cause the skin to be tight, smooth, and shiny.
Pallor, cool skin at edematous area	Excess fluid causes a decrease in circulation. The skin becomes pale, shiny, and cool.
Puffy eyelids (periorbital edema)	Swollen eyelids occur with generalized edema.
Weight gain	A gain of 2.2 pounds is equivalent to a gain of 1 liter of body water.

continues on the following page

Table 2-3

(Continued)

Signs and Symptoms	Rationale
Laboratory Tests	
Decreased serum osmolality	Excess fluid dilutes solute concentration; thus, serum osmolality is below 280 mOsm/kg.
Decreased serum protein and albumin, BUN, Hgb, Hct	Serum protein, albumin, BUN, and Hgb and Hct levels can be decreased due to excess fluid volume (hemodilution).
Increased CVP (central venous pressure)	An increase in CVP measurement of more than 12–15 cm H_2O is indicative of hypervolemia, evidenced as an increase in the fluid pressure.

Table 2-4

Basic Management for ECFVE or Edema

Correction Measures	Rationale
Diuretics: thiazides, high ceiling (loop)	Potassium-wasting diuretics are potent and promote the loss of sodium, water, and unfortunately, potassium. Diuretics cause a decrease in fluid volume excess via kidneys.
Digoxin	This cardiac glycoside causes the heart to beat more forcefully; thus, it improves heart function and circulation. Increased circulation promotes water loss through the kidneys.
Diet	A diet low in sodium decreases sodium and water retention.
Increased protein intake for a malnourished person	Protein increases the oncotic pressure in the vessels, thus pulling water out of the tissues.

3. A constant, irritated cough is frequently the first clinical symptom of hypervolemia. It is caused by excess fluid "backed up" into the lungs.

4. For quick assessment of ECFVE, check for hand vein engorgement. If the peripheral veins in the hand remain engorged when the hand is elevated above the heart level for 10 seconds, ECFVE or hypervolemia is present.

5. Moist rales in the lung usually indicate that the lungs are congested with fluid.

6. Peripheral edema present in the morning may result from inadequate heart, liver, or kidney function. Peripheral edema in the evening may be due to fluid stasis—dependent edema. Peripheral edema should be assessed in the morning before the client gets out of bed.

7. A weight gain of 2.2 pounds is equivalent to the retention of 1 liter of body water.

8. Excess fluid dilutes solute concentration in the vascular space. A serum osmolality of <280 mOsm/kg indicates an ECFVE.

▶ CLIENT MANAGEMENT

Assessment

- Obtain a client history to identify typical health problems that may contribute to the development of ECFVE, such as congestive heart failure (CHF), kidney or liver disease, infection, and malnutrition.

- Obtain a dietary history that emphasizes sodium, protein, and water intake.

- Assess vital signs and urinary output. Report a bounding pulse.

- Check client's weight. Present weight is a baseline for comparison with daily weight.

- Assess for signs and symptoms of hypervolemia: constant, irritated cough, dyspnea, neck and hand vein engorgement, chest rales.

- Check laboratory test results; a decreased hematocrit and hemoglobin level that had previously been normal may indicate ECFVE. Serum sodium levels may or may not be elevated because of hemodilution.

- Assess urine output; decreased urinary output may be a sign of body fluid retention and/or renal dysfunction.

- Auscultate the lungs for diminished breath sound and rales, which could be due to pulmonary edema.

- Assess extremities for peripheral edema. Assessment for pitting edema in the lower extremities should be performed in the morning before the client arises.
- Make a quick assessment for hypervolemia by checking the peripheral veins in the hand, first lowering the hand and then raising the hand above the heart level.

Diagnoses

- *Fluid Volume Excess, Edema,* related to body fluid overload secondary to heart, renal, or liver dysfunction
- *Ineffective Breathing Pattern,* related to increased capillary permeability causing fluid overload in the lung tissue (pulmonary edema)
- *Altered Tissue Perfusion: Decreased,* related to hypervolemia as manifested by peripheral edema

Interventions

- Monitor vital signs with particular attention to respiratory status. Report abnormal findings, i.e., rales, diminished breath sound.
- Monitor weight daily before breakfast. A weight gain of 2.2 pounds (1 kg) is equivalent to 1 liter of water. Usually edema does not occur unless there are 2 or more liters of excess body fluids.
- Monitor diet. Instruct the client to avoid excess use of salt on foods. Sodium retains water.
- Observe for the presence or decline of edema on a daily basis. Check for pitted edema in the morning.
- Check laboratory test results that are pertinent to electrolyte status and fluid balance.
- Monitor urine output. Urine output should be at least 250 mL per 8 hours.
- Administer diuretics as ordered. Assess fluid and electrolyte balance.
- Listen to client's concerns. Answer questions or refer questions to appropriate health professionals.

Evaluation/Outcome

- Evaluate that the cause of extracellular fluid volume excess (ECFVE) has been controlled or eliminated.

- Remain free of signs and symptoms of overhydration/hypervolemia; dyspnea, neck vein engorgement, moist rales in the lung, and peripheral edema are absent.

- Evaluate the effects of clinical management for ECFVE; pulmonary edema and/or peripheral edema are absent or decreased because of clinical management.

- Urine output is increased to baseline measurement; vital signs are within normal range.

- Maintain a patent airway and the breath sounds are improved.

- Determine that the serum electrolytes are within normal range.

Extracellular Fluid Volume Shift (ECFVS)

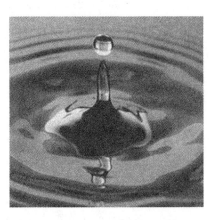

▌ INTRODUCTION

In the extracellular fluid compartment, ECF is constantly shifting between the intravascular and interstitial spaces for the purpose of maintaining fluid balance. When fluid volume with electrolytes and protein shifts from the intravascular to the interstitial spaces and remains there, this fluid is referred to as **third-space fluid.** This fluid is nonfunctional and is considered to be physiologically useless. Later, third-space fluid shifts back from the interstitial space to the intravascular space.

▌ PATHOPHYSIOLOGY

Refer to the Pathophysiology section in Chapters 1 (ECFVD) and 2 (ECFVE).

▌ ETIOLOGY

Clinical causes of ECFV shift can be as simple as a blister or sprain or as serious as massive injuries, burns, ascites, abdominal surgery, a perforated peptic ulcer, intestinal obstruction, or severe infections. Burns, massive injuries, and abdominal surgery are the most common causes of third-space fluid.

Fluid shift occurs in two phases. The first phase is when fluid shifts from the intravascular to the interstitial (vessel/plasma to tissue) space. For example, with burns, fluid loss occurs at the burned area and surrounding tissues. Fluid from the vascular space "pours" into the burned site and remains there for 3–5 days. When massive amounts of fluid shift to the tissues and remain there, fluid in the vascular space decreases and hypovolemia occurs. In the second phase of fluid shift, fluid then shifts from the injured tissue space back to the vascular space (vessels); hypervolemia may result. Table 3-1 presents the two phases of fluid volume shift, causes, approximate times for occurrence, and possible resulting type of fluid imbalance.

▶ CLINICAL MANIFESTATIONS

In a fluid shift due to tissue injury, it takes approximately 24–48 hours for the fluid to leave the blood vessels and accumulate in the injured tissue spaces. Edema may or may not be visible. When fluid (massive amounts) shifts out of the vessels, changes in vital signs occur that are similar to symptoms of shock. Vital sign measures are similar to those of a fluid volume deficit (marked dehydration). These measures include increased pulse rate, increased respiration, and decreased systolic blood pressure

Table 3-1

Fluid Volume Shift

Phase	Fluid Shift	Cause	Time Occurrence	Resulting Type of Fluid Imbalance
I	Intravascular (vessel) to the interstitial (tissue) spaces	*Minor:* blister, sprain *Major:* burns, abdominal surgery, intestinal obstruction, crushing wounds, severe infections	24–48 h	Hypovolemia
II	Interstitial to intravascular spaces		3–5 days	Hypervolemia

(depending on the severity of fluid loss to the injured site). Other shock-like symptoms include cold extremities, pallor, confusion, and disorientation. In severe cases the hemoglobin and hematocrit can be increased.

After 3–5 days following severe tissue injury, fluid shifts from the injured site to the vascular space or blood vessels. If the kidneys cannot excrete the excess fluid from the vascular space, ECFVE or hypervolemia results. Symptoms related to intravascular overload include constant, irritated cough, dyspnea, moist chest rales, full bounding pulse, and hand and neck vein engorgement. Table 3-2 lists the two phases of fluid shifts, signs and symptoms, and fluid correction ratio.

▶ CLINICAL MANAGEMENT

An assessment must be completed in order to determine the cause of the third-space fluid. If the cause is due to a minor injury such as a sprain or blisters, the amount of fluid shift is usually minor. Ice packs applied periodically to the sprained area can decrease the amount of fluid shift during the first 24 hours. Fluid replacement is not necessary. However, when there is severe tissue destruction, the fluid shift may be so severe that hypovolemia results from the massive amount of fluid shifting from the vascular space into the injured tissue areas. During the first phase of fluid shift to the injured tissue site, intravenous (IV) infusion in

Table 3-2

ECFV Shift: Signs, Symptoms, and Corrections

Phase of Fluid Shift	Signs and Symptoms	Fluid Correction Ratio
Phase 1	*Shock-like Symptoms—* Severe ECFVD Pulse, respiration, BP Cold, clammy skin, pallor, confusion, disorientation	*IV Intake to Urine Output* 3 : 1 Three times more IV intake to urine output
Phase 2	*Overhydration-like Symptoms* Constant, irritated cough, dyspnea, bounding pulse, vein engorgement, moist chest rales	*IV Intake to Urine Output* 1 : 3 One to three ratio: IV intake to urine output

the amount of two to three times the urine output may be necessary to maintain the circulating fluid volume. The ratio is three times the intake to one time the output.

During the second phase of fluid shift, less IV fluid is needed. This fluid reduction is because a large quantity of fluid shifts back into the vascular space, and too much IV fluid may cause a fluid overload. In the second phase of fluid shift with normal renal function, the urine output increases. Excreting excess fluid prevents fluid overload. The amount of IV fluid administered should decrease by a ratio of 1 : 3 (one time the intake to three times the urine output) (see Table 3-2).

▶ CLIENT MANAGEMENT

Assessment

For extracellular fluid volume shift, refer to Chapter 1 (ECFVD) and Chapter 2 (ECFVE).

Diagnoses

For extracellular fluid volume shift, refer to Chapter 1 (ECFVD) and Chapter 2 (ECFVE).

Interventions

For extracellular fluid volume shift, refer to Chapter 1 (ECFVD) and Chapter 2 (ECFVE).

Evaluation/Outcome

For extracellular fluid volume shift, refer to Chapter 1 (ECFVD) and Chapter 2 (ECFVE).

Intracellular Fluid Volume Excess (ICFVE)

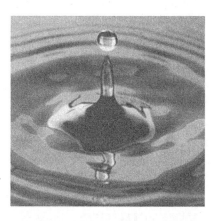

▌ INTRODUCTION

Intracellular fluid volume excess (ICFVE), also referred to as water intoxication, results from an excess of water or a decrease in the solute concentration in the intravascular system. Fluid in the blood vessels is hypo-osmolar. As a result of this excess water, the serum osmolality is decreased.

Hypo-osmolar fluid (decreased solute concentration in the circulating vascular fluid) moves by the process of osmosis from areas of lesser concentration of solutes to areas of greater concentration of solutes. Since intracellular fluid (cells) is iso-osmolar, the hypo-osmolar fluid from the vascular space moves into the cells.

▌ PATHOPHYSIOLOGY

In ICFVE, the cerebral cells are usually the first cells involved in the fluid shift from the vascular to the cellular space. As fluid shifts into the cells, the cells swell, causing cellular edema. An excess secretion of the antidiuretic hormone (ADH) causes water to be reabsorbed from the renal tubules. This results in an increase in diluted fluid volume (hypo-osmolar vascular fluid), which causes additional fluid to move from the vascular space into the cells, causing cerebral edema.

Edema may result from an excess of sodium, whereas water intoxication results from an excess of water. With edema there is excessive fluid in the extracellular fluid compartment, and with water intoxication (ICFVE) there is excess fluid in the intracellular fluid compartment. Edema is the accumulation of fluid in the interstitial spaces, and water intoxication is the excess of hypo-osmolar fluid in the vessels moving into the cells. Figure 4-1 shows the differences between the two fluid imbalances, ECFVE and ICFVE.

▌ ETIOLOGY

Intracellular fluid volume excess is not as common as ECFVD and ECFVE, but if untreated, it can cause serious health problems. Common causes of water intoxication are the intake of water-free solutes and the administration of hypo-osmolar intravenous fluids such as 0.45% sodium chloride ($\frac{1}{2}$ normal saline solution) and 5% dextrose in water

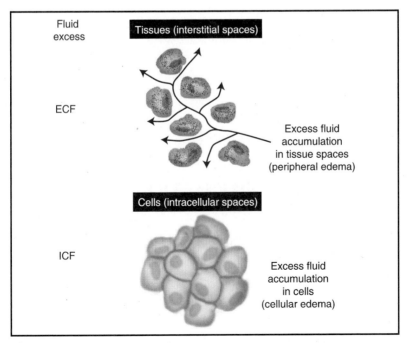

Figure 4-1 Fluid Excess in ECF and ICF Compartments

(D₅W). Dextrose 5% in water is an iso-osmolar IV solution; however, the dextrose is metabolized quickly, leaving water or a hypo-osmolar solution.

There are four major conditions that may cause ICFVE:

1. Excessive nonsolute water intake
2. Solute deficit (electrolyte and protein)
3. Increased secretion of the antidiuretic hormone (ADH)
4. Kidney dysfunction (inability to excrete excess water)

Table 4-1 lists four major conditions and laboratory tests for ICFVE, their causes, and rationale.

It is difficult for a person to drink himself or herself into intracellular fluid volume excess or water intoxication unless the renal mechanisms for elimination fail or psychogenic polydipsia occurs. If excessive water has been given and the kidneys are not functioning properly, water retention and water intoxication are likely to occur.

The most common occurrence of ICFVE is seen in postoperative clients when oral and intravenous fluids have been forced without compensatory amounts of salt. In these situations, the amount of water taken in exceeds that which the kidneys excrete. A postoperative client receiving several liters of 5% dextrose in water, ice chips, and sips of water by mouth can develop water intoxication (ICFVE). The dextrose in D₅W is metabolized rapidly and the solution in the vascular space becomes hypo-osmolar. After major surgery, there is frequently an overproduction of the antidiuretic hormone (ADH), known as the syndrome of inappropriate ADH secretions (SIADH). This is partly due to tissue trauma, anesthesia, pain, and narcotics. Because of SIADH, water excretion decreases, causing the urine volume to drop and the vascular fluid volume to increase. The vascular fluid is mainly hypo-osmolar; this diluted vascular fluid moves to the cells that have a higher solute concentration, thus water intoxication results.

▶ CLINICAL MANIFESTATIONS

An early sign/symptom of ICFVE is headaches. As the hypo-osmolar body fluids continue to pass into cerebral cells, the swollen cerebral cells cause behavioral changes such as apprehension, irritability, confusion, and disorientation. The intracranial pressure is increased. With progressive intracellular fluid volume excess, the blood pressure increases, pulse rate decreases, and respirations increase. The clinical signs, symptoms, and rationale of ICFVE are explained in Table 4-2.

Table 4-1

Causes of Intracellular Fluid Volume Excess: Water Intoxication

Conditions	Causes	Rationale
Excessive water intake	Excessive plain water intake	Water intake with few or no solutes dilutes the vascular fluid.
	Continuous use of IV hypo-osmolar solutions (0.45% saline, D_5W)	Overuse of hypo-osmolar solutions can cause hypo-osmolar vascular fluid. Dextrose is metabolized rapidly, leaving water.
	Psychogenic polydipsia	Compulsive drinking of plain water can result in water intoxication.
Solute deficit	Diet low in electrolytes and protein	Decrease in electrolytes and protein may cause hypo-osmolar vascular fluids.
	Irrigation of nasogastric tube with water (not saline)	GI tract is rich in electrolytes. Plain water can wash out the electrolytes.
	Plain water enema	Plain water can wash out the electrolytes.
Excess ADH secretion	Stress, surgery, drugs (narcotics, anesthesia), pain, and tumors (brain, lung)	Overproduction of ADH is known as secretion (syndrome) of inappropriate antidiuretic hormone (SIADH), which causes mass amounts of water reabsorption by the kidneys and results in hypo-osmolar fluids.
	Brain injury or tumor	Cerebral cell injury may increase ADH production, causing excessive water reabsorption.
Kidney dysfunction	Renal impairment	Kidney dysfunction can decrease water excretion.
Abnormal laboratory tests	Decreased serum sodium level and decreased serum osmolality	Because of hemodilution, the solutes in the vascular fluid are decreased in proportion to water.

Table 4-2

Clinical Signs and Symptoms of Intracellular Fluid Volume Excess—Water Intoxication

Type of Symptoms	Signs and Symptoms	Rationale
Early	Headache Nausea and vomiting Excessive perspiration Acute weight gain	Cerebral cells absorb hypo-osmolar fluid more quickly than other cells.

Progressive
Central nervous system (CNS)
	Behavioral changes:
	  progressive apprehension,
	  irritability, disorientation,
	  confusion
	Drowsiness, Incoordination
	Blurred vision
	Elevated intracranial pressure
	  (ICP)
		Hypo-osmolar body fluids usually pass into cerebral cells first. Swollen cerebral cells can cause behavioral changes and elevate ICP.

Vital signs (VS)	Blood pressure ↑ Bradycardia (slow pulse rate) Respiration ↑	VS are the opposite of shock. VS are similar to those in increased ICP.
Later (CNS)	Neuroexcitability (muscle twitching) Projectile vomiting Papilledema Delirium Convulsions, then coma	Severe CNS changes occur when water intoxication is not corrected.
Skin	Warm, moist, and flushed	

❙ CLINICAL MANAGEMENT

The overall objectives for clinical management of ICFVE are to reduce excess water intake and to promote water excretion. In less severe cases, water restriction may be sufficient or an extracellular replacement solution such as lactated Ringer's or normal saline solution can increase the osmolality of the extracellular fluid. A concentrated saline solution (3%) may be given in severe cases of water intoxication in order to raise the extracellular electrolyte concentration in order to draw the water out of the intracellular space and increase urine output.

However, administration of additional salt to a person who already has too much water can expand the blood volume and the interstitial

Table 4-3

Clinical Management for Clients Having ICFVE

Stage of ICFVE	Corrective Measures
Early stage	Restrict plain water intake and ice chips. Administer balanced electrolyte solution (BES) such as lactated Ringer's solution, normal saline solution, 5% dextrose in 0.45% normal saline solution. Avoid using only 5% dextrose in water.
Moderate stage without severe behavioral changes	Same as the early stage. Five percent dextrose in 0.9% NaCl may be needed.
Moderate to severe stage with behavioral changes and elevated intracranial pressure (ICP)	Restrict plain water intake and ice chips. Discontinue 5% dextrose in water for replacement therapy. Administer concentrated saline (3%) solution and monitor for fluid overload. Administer osmotic diuretic such as mannitol.

fluid resulting in edema. An osmotic diuretic induces diuresis and promotes the loss of retained fluid, especially from the cells. Table 4-3 lists the methods in promoting water excretion for correcting ICFVE.

● Clinical Considerations: ICFVE

1. ICFVE is also known as water intoxication—excess water in the cells. It usually results from an excess of hypo-osmolar (hypotonic) vascular fluid. Water intoxication is not the same as edema. Edema usually results from sodium retention, whereas water intoxication results from excess water.

2. In ICFVE, cerebral cells are usually the first cells involved in the fluid shift from the vascular to the cellular (cell) space. Large amounts of fluid shifting into the cerebral cells can result in cerebral edema.

3. Continuous administration of intravenous solutions that are hypotonic or the continuous use of 5% dextrose in water can result in ICFVE. In the latter case, dextrose is metabolized rapidly in the body; thus water remains. At least 1 or 2 liters of the dextrose solution should contain a percentage of a saline solution or be administered in combination with solutes such as lactated Ringer's.

4. Headache, nausea, and vomiting are early signs and symptoms of ICFVE. As ICFVE progresses, behavioral changes such as irritability,

disorientation, and confusion may occur. Drowsiness and blurred vision may result.

5. Changes in vital signs are similar to those of cerebral edema: increased blood pressure, decreased pulse rate, and increased respirations.

6. A concentrated saline solution (3% NaCl) can be administered for severe ICFVE. It is given if the serum sodium is less than 115 mEq/L. Also, it draws the water out of the swollen cells.

7. Water restriction is suggested for mild ICFVE.

▶ CLIENT MANAGEMENT

Assessment

- Obtain a history to identify the possible cause(s) of ICFVE such as continuous use of D_5W without solutes (saline), excessive intake of oral fluid without solutes, or major surgical procedure that might cause SIADH.

- Assess vital signs (VS) by obtaining a baseline of VS that can be compared with past and future VS. Note the VS typical for cerebral edema, i.e., increased blood pressure, decreased pulse rate, and increased respirations.

- Assess for behavioral changes, such as apprehension, irritability, confusion, and/or disorientation. Headache is an early symptom of ICFVE.

- Assess for weight changes. With ICFVE, there is usually an acute weight gain; however, with peripheral edema, the weight gain occurs more slowly.

Diagnoses

- *Fluid Volume Excess, Water Intoxication,* related to excessive ingestion and infusion of hypo-osmolar fluids and solutions, and major surgical procedure causing SIADH

- *Risk for Injury,* related to confusion from cerebral edema secondary to ICFVE

Interventions

- Monitor fluid replacement. Report if the client is receiving ONLY 5% dextrose in water continuously without any solutes such as sodium chloride.

- Offer fluids that contain solutes to the postoperative client. Giving only plain water and ice chips increases the hypo-osmolar state.

- Monitor urine output. This is especially important postoperatively.

- Monitor vital signs and observe for behavioral changes.

- Protect the client from injury during periods of confusion and disorientation.

- Listen to client's and family's concerns. Refer unknown answers to appropriate health professionals.

Evaluation/Outcome

- Evaluate that the cause of intracellular fluid volume excess (ICFVE) has been corrected or controlled.

- Remain free of signs and symptoms of ICFVE or water intoxication; vital signs return to normal ranges, headaches have been lessened or absent.

- Evaluate the effects of clinical management of ICFVE; hypotonic/hypo-osmolar solutions discontinued, solutes offered with fluids.

- Responds clearly without confusion.

Electrolytes and Their Influence on the Body

▶ INTRODUCTION

Chemical compounds develop a tiny electrical charge when dissolved in water. The compounds break into separate particles known as ions; this process is referred to as ionization, and the compounds are known as electrolytes. Some electrolytes develop a positive charge (cations) when placed in water; others develop a negative charge (anions).

In this unit, six electrolytes [potassium, sodium, chloride, calcium, magnesium, and phosphorus (phosphate)] are discussed in relation to basic information associated with each electrolyte in terms of pathophysiology, etiology, clinical manifestations, and clinical management issues. Health assessment and intervention guidelines follow the presentation of each electrolyte.

▶ ELECTROLYTES: CATION AND ANION

Electrolytes are compounds that, when placed in solution, conduct an electric current and emit dissociated particles of electrolytes (ions) that carry either a positive charge (cation) or a negative charge (anion). Table U2-1 gives the principal cations and anions in human body fluids. Note the symbols for each electrolyte (e.g., K, Na) and their charge ($^+$ and $^-$).

The term *milliequivalents* is used to express the number of ionic charges of each electrolyte. Serum electrolyte values are expressed in milliequivalents and milligrams. The milliequivalents of electrolytes are the chemical activity of the ion rather than their weight. Table U2-2 gives the weights and equivalences of four cations and an anion. Note how the weights of the named ions differ but the equivalences remain the same according to their ionic charge.

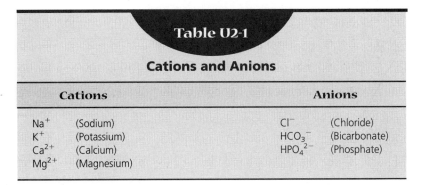

Table U2-1

Cations and Anions

Cations		Anions	
Na^+	(Sodium)	Cl^-	(Chloride)
K^+	(Potassium)	HCO_3^-	(Bicarbonate)
Ca^{2+}	(Calcium)	HPO_4^{2-}	(Phosphate)
Mg^{2+}	(Magnesium)		

Table U2-2

Electrolyte Equivalents

Ion	Weight (mg)	Equivalence (mEq)
Na^+	23	1
K^+	39	1
Cl^-	35	1
Ca^{++}	40	2
Mg^{++}	24	2

The electrolyte composition of fluid differs within the two main classes of body fluid (intracellular fluid and the extracellular fluid); refer to Unit I. Table U2-3 gives the ion concentrations of the intravascular fluid (referred to as plasma), interstitial fluid, and intracellular fluid. Note that sodium (Na) is more plentiful in the extracellular fluid (plasma and interstitial fluid) and potassium (K) is more plentiful in the intracellular fluid. Figure U2-1 shows the various cations and anions in extracellular and intracellular fluids.

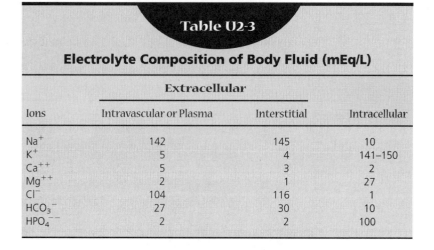

Table U2-3

Electrolyte Composition of Body Fluid (mEq/L)

	Extracellular		Intracellular
Ions	Intravascular or Plasma	Interstitial	
Na^+	142	145	10
K^+	5	4	141–150
Ca^{++}	5	3	2
Mg^{++}	2	1	27
Cl^-	104	116	1
HCO_3^-	27	30	10
HPO_4^{--}	2	2	100

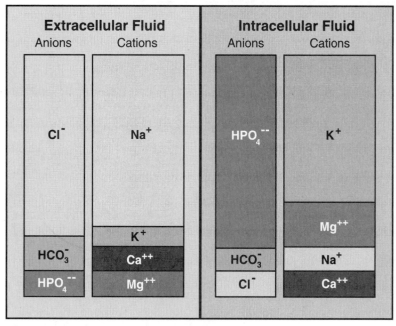

Figure U2-1 Anions and Cations in Body Fluid

Potassium Imbalances

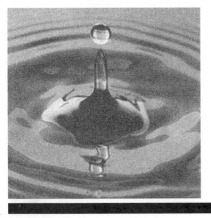

▶ INTRODUCTION

Potassium (K), a cation, is the most abundant cation in the body cells. Ninety-seven percent of the body's potassium is found in the intracellular fluid (ICF) and 2–3% is found in the extracellular fluid (ECF), which comprises of intravascular (in vessels) and interstitial fluids (between tissues). Potassium is also plentiful in the gastrointestinal tract. The potassium level in the cells is approximately 150 mEq, and the potassium level in the ECF is 3.5–5.3 mEq. Because potassium levels cannot be measured within the cells, the potassium level is monitored by obtaining intravascular fluid or blood plasma specimens.

The normal plasma/serum potassium range is narrow; therefore, a serum potassium level outside the normal range may be life threatening. A serum potassium level less than 2.5 mEq/L or greater than 7.0 mEq/L can cause cardiac arrest. Thus, serum potassium values need to be closely monitored.

Basic information related to potassium balance is summarized in Table 5-1. Deviations from the normal result in a potassium imbalance.

Table 5-1

Basic Information Related to Potassium Balance

Categories	Potassium Data
Distribution	Ninety-seven percent of potassium is located within the cells (intracellular fluid). Two to 3% of potassium is located within the extracellular fluid. Potassium is most plentiful in the GI tract.
Functions	Potassium (1) promotes the transmission and conduction of nerve impulses and the contraction of skeletal, cardiac, and smooth muscles; (2) assists in the regulation of intracellular osmolality; (3) promotes enzyme action for cellular metabolism; and (4) assists in maintenance acid-base balance. A potassium deficit is associated with alkalosis and a potassium excess is related to acidosis.
Normal serum value	3.5–5.3 mEq/L. A potassium deficit (hypokalemia) is less than 3.5 mEq/L and a potassium excess (hyperkalemia) is greater than 5.3 mEq/L.
Normal potassium excretion (urine)	Twenty to 120 mEq of potassium per day is excreted by the kidneys.
Food sources	Foods rich in potassium include vegetables, fruits, dry fruits, nuts, and meat. Foods rich in sodium promote a potassium loss.
Dietary requirements	Normal daily potassium intake is 40–60 mEq. Potassium is poorly stored in the body, so a daily potassium intake is essential.
Excretion	Eighty to 90% of the body's potassium is excreted through the kidneys. Ten to 20% is excreted in the feces.

❱ PATHOPHYSIOLOGY

The assimilative processes involved in the formation of new tissue are referred to as **anabolism,** and the reactions concerned with tissue breakdown are referred to as **catabolism.** When cellular activity is anabolic (building up), potassium enters the cells. When cellular activity is catabolic (breaking down), potassium leaves the cells. When tissues are destroyed as a result of trauma, starvation, or wasting diseases, large quantities of potassium leave the cells. If the kidneys are functioning, potassium is excreted and hypokalemia results. The pathophysiology related to potassium loss and retention is summarized in Table 5-2.

During exercise, when muscles contract, the cells lose potassium and absorb a nearly equal quantity of sodium from the extracellular fluid. After exercise, when the muscles are recovering from fatigue, potassium reenters the cells and most of the sodium returns to the extracellular

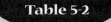

Table 5-2

Pathophysiology Related to Potassium Loss and Retention

Potassium Imbalance	Pathophysiology
Potassium loss	*Cellular Potassium Loss*
	Tissue injury: trauma, malnutrition
	Muscle contraction: continuous or strenuous exercise
	GI losses: vomiting, diarrhea
	Hormonal Influence
	Aldosterone promotes sodium retention and potassium excretion.
	Insulin promotes potassium leaving the ECF and moving into cells.
	Renal Potassium Loss
	Normal kidney function excretes excess potassium from the ECF.
Potassium retention	*Renal Dysfunction*
	Decreased renal function causes a buildup of potassium in the ECF, resulting in hyperkalemia.

fluid. The cations potassium and sodium have an opposing effect on each other in the extracellular fluid. When one is retained, the other is excreted.

Hormonal influences affect serum potassium levels. Physiologic or psychologic stress causes a release of an excessive amount of potassium that is then lost through the kidneys. This potassium loss depletes the cells' supply. Stress also stimulates the adrenal gland to overproduce **aldosterone,** an adrenal cortical hormone. This hormone influences the kidneys to excrete potassium and to retain sodium, chloride, and water.

Insulin production or administration promotes glucose and potassium uptake by the cells and thus decreases the serum potassium level. Insulin administration may be used to temporarily correct a mild hyperkalemic state by forcing the potassium back into the cells. It is believed that glucagon increases the serum potassium level by releasing potassium from the liver and muscle cells.

When renal function is normal, the excess potassium is slowly excreted by the kidneys. However, if potassium intake is decreased without oral or intravenous supplements, potassium excretion by the kidneys can lead to potassium depletion or hypokalemia. If the kidneys are injured or diseased and the urine output is markedly decreased, potassium concentration increases in the extracellular fluid and hyperkalemia results.

▶ ETIOLOGY

Daily potassium intake is necessary because potassium is poorly conserved within the body. Inadequate intake through a balanced diet may result in a potassium deficit. The elderly and the young tend to lose potassium faster than healthy adults; thus the potassium level must be monitored closely.

Causes of hypokalemia include dietary changes, gastrointestinal losses, renal losses, hormonal influence, and cellular damage. Summary data of these losses are presented in Table 5-3. Causes of hyperkalemia include excessive potassium intake, decreased renal function, altered cellular function, hormonal deficiency, and pseudohyperkalemia. Summary data are presented in Table 5-4.

▶ CLINICAL MANIFESTATIONS

Clinical manifestations of hypokalemia and hyperkalemia can be determined by the serum potassium level, electrocardiography (ECG/EKG) tracings, and specific signs and symptoms related to gastrointestinal, cardiac, renal, and neurologic abnormalities. The serum potassium level and the ECG play a critical role in determining the severity of the potassium imbalance. Mild hypokalemia may go undetected until the serum potassium level is less than 3.2 mEq/L. Signs and symptoms of hyperkalemia may not be noted until the serum potassium level exceeds 5.6 mEq/L.

A potassium deficit slows muscular contraction; thus skeletal muscle contraction and GI smooth muscle activity are slowed. Hypokalemia decreases GI motility, which when severe may result in a paralytic ileus.

Mild to moderate hyperkalemia causes muscle irritability, while severe hyperkalemia causes muscle weakness. When a serum potassium level reaches 6.0 mEq/L, paresthesia (numbness, tingling) and an increased heart rate may be apparent. Table 5-5 lists specific signs and symptoms indicative of hypokalemia and hyperkalemia.

Potassium is abundant in cardiac muscle, and a deficit may result in cardiac dysrhythmias. Common ECG changes associated with hypokalemia include premature ventricular contractions (PVCs), a flat or inverted T wave, and a depressed ST segment. Figure 5-1 (see page 52) displays the ECG results related to hypokalemia, and Figure 5-2 (see page 53) includes the ECG changes resulting from hyperkalemia. A serum potassium level >6.0 mEq/L causes the myocardium to become flaccid and dilate; an atrial or ventricular dysrhythmia is likely to occur. ECG changes

Table 5-3

Causes of Hypokalemia (Serum Potassium Deficit)

Etiology	Rationale
Dietary Changes Malnutrition, starvation, alcoholism, unbalanced reducing diets, anorexia nervosa, crash diets	Potassium is poorly conserved in the body. For a potassium deficit to occur, a prolonged, inadequate potassium intake must occur.
Gastrointestinal Losses Vomiting, diarrhea, gastric/intestinal suctioning, intestinal fistula, laxative abuse, bulimia, enemas	Potassium is plentiful in the GI tract. With the loss of GI secretions, large amounts of potassium ions are lost.
Renal Losses Diuretics, diuretic phase of acute renal failure, hemodialysis and peritoneal dialysis	The kidneys excrete 80–90% of the potassium lost. Diuretics are the major cause of hypokalemia, especially potassium-wasting diuretics [thiazides, loop (high-ceiling), osmotic]
Hormonal Influence Steroids, Cushing's syndrome, stress, excessive intake of licorice	Steroids, especially cortisone and aldosterone, promote potassium excretion and sodium retention. Stress increases the production of steroids in the body. In Cushing's syndrome, there is an excess production of adrenocortical hormones (corticol and aldosterone). Licorice contains glyceric acid, which has an aldosteronelike effect.
Cellular Damage Trauma, tissue injury, surgery, burns	Cellular and tissue damage cause potassium to be released in the intravascular fluid. More potassium is needed to repair injured tissue.
Redistribution of Potassium Insulin, alkalotic state	Insulin moves glucose and potassium i̶ cells. Metabolic alkalosis pr᷑ movement of potassium i̶

Table 5-4

Causes of Hyperkalemia (Serum Potassium Excess)

Etiology	Rationale
Excessive Potassium Intake	
Oral potassium supplements	A potassium consumption rate greater than the potassium excretion rate increases the serum potassium level.
IV potassium infusions	Adequate urinary output must be determined when giving a potassium supplement.
Decreased Renal Function	
Acute renal failure	Because potassium is generally excreted in the urine,
Chronic renal failure	anuria and oliguria cause a potassium buildup in the plasma.
Potassium-sparing diuretics	Potassium-sparing diuretics can cause an aldosterone deficiency, promoting potassium retention.
Altered Cellular Function	
Severe traumatic injury	Cellular injury increases potassium loss due to cell breakdown. Potassium excretion may be greater than cellular K reabsorption. Potassium can accumulate in the plasma.
Metabolic acidosis	In acidosis, the hydrogen ion moves into the cells and potassium moves out of the cells, increasing the serum potassium level.
Blood for transfusion that is 1–3 weeks old	As stored blood for transfusion ages, hemolysis (breakdown of red blood cells) occurs; potassium from the cells is released into the ECF.
Hormonal Deficiency	
Addison's disease	Reduced secretion of the adrenocortical hormones causes a retention of potassium and a loss of sodium.
Pseudohyperkalemia	
Hemolysis	With hemolysis, ruptured red blood cells release potassium into the ECF.
Tourniquet application	A tourniquet that has been applied too tightly or
Phlebotomy	rapidly drawing blood with a small needle lumen (<21 gauge) can cause a falsely elevated potassium level in the blood specimen.

Table 5-5

Clinical Manifestations of Potassium Imbalances

Body Involvement	Hypokalemia	Hyperkalemia
Gastrointestinal Abnormalities	*Anorexia Nausea *Vomiting Diarrhea †Abdominal distention †Decreased peristalsis or silent ileus	*Nausea *Diarrhea †Abdominal cramps
Cardiac Abnormalities	†Dysrhythmias †Vertigo Cardiac arrest when severe	Tachycardia, later †bradycardia, and finally cardiac arrest (severe)
ECG/EKG	†Flat or inverted T wave Depressed ST segment	†Peaked, narrow T wave Shortened QT interval Prolonged PR interval followed by disappearance of P wave Prolonged QRS interval if level continues to rise
Renal Abnormalities	Polyuria	†Oliguria or anuria
Neuromuscular Abnormalities	†Malaise Drowsiness †Muscular weakness Confusion Mental depression Diminished deep tendon reflexes Respiratory paralysis	Weakness, numbness, or tingling sensation Muscle cramps
Laboratory Values Serum potassium	<3.5 mEq/L	>5.3 mEq/L

†Most commonly seen symptoms of hypo-hyperkalemia
*Commonly seen symptoms of hypo-hyperkalemia

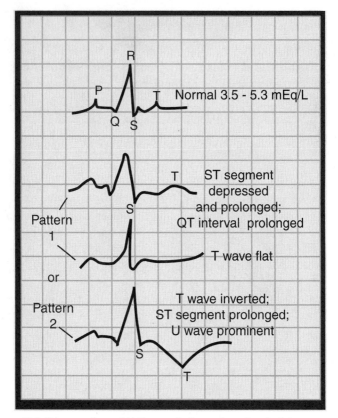

Figure 5-1 Electrocardiographic Changes in Serum Potassium Deficit

usually do not occur until the serum potassium level approaches 7.0 mEq/L. ECG findings for hyperkalemia include narrow peaked T waves, a widened QRS complex, a depressed ST segment, and a widened PR interval. These heart changes result in a decreased cardiac output.

▶ CLINICAL MANAGEMENT

Successful clinical management of a potassium imbalance requires immediate intervention if the potassium is less than 3.0 mEq/L or more than 5.8 mEq/L. Oral potassium replacement therapy is frequently ordered for a mild potassium deficit (3.3–3.4 mEq/L) or for preventive purposes. Potassium is irritating to the GI tract and should be ingested with at least 6–8 ounces of fluid. Intravenous (IV) potassium chloride (KCl) is suggested for a moderate to severe potassium deficit (<3.2 q/L). Intravenous KCl should NEVER be administered as a bolus or IV

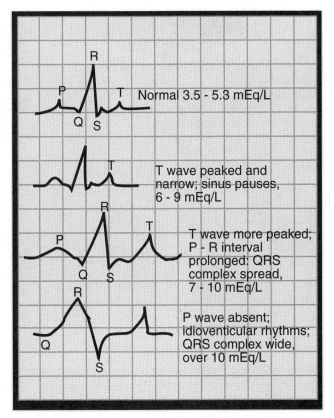

Figure 5-2 Electrocardiographic Changes in Serum Potassium Concentration

push. Cardiac arrest can result. Intravenous KCl must be well diluted in an IV solution. Table 5-6 lists selected potassium replacement drugs. Serum levels of magnesium, chloride, and protein should be checked when correcting hypokalemia. Low values of Mg, Cl, and protein can inhibit potassium utilization by the body.

Temporary interventions to correct hyperkalemia include the use of sodium bicarbonate and insulin and glucose infusion. These agents initially move potassium back into the cells; however, if the drugs are repeated for the purpose of decreasing the potassium level, they may not be effective. Calcium gluconate infusions may be prescribed to decrease the antagonistic effect of potassium excess on the myocardium when the cardiac disturbance is due to hyperkalemia.

With severe hyperkalemia (>6.8 mEq/L), polystyrene sulfonate (Kayexalate), a cation exchange resin, may be given orally or rectally. A potassium ion is exchanged for a sodium ion in the intestinal tract, and

Table 5-6

Oral Potassium Supplements

Preparation	Drug
Liquid	Potassium chloride 10% = 20 mEq/15 mL; 20% = 40 mEq/15 mL Kay Ciel (potassium chloride) Kaochlor 10% (potassium chloride) Kaon Cl 20 (potassium chloride) Potassium Triplex (potassium acetate, bicarbonate, citrate)
Tablet/capsule	Potassium chloride (enteric-coated tablet) Kaon—plain (potassium gluconate) Kaon Cl (potassium chloride) Slow K (potassium chloride—8 mEq) Kaochlor (potassium chloride) K-Lyte—plain (potassium bicarbonate-effervescent tablet) K-Lyte/Cl (potassium chloride)

the potassium ion is excreted in the stool. Because Kayexalate is constipating, sorbitol may be given with Kayexalate to prevent constipation and induce diarrhea. A retention enema is the mode for administering rectal Kayexalate and sorbitol. Table 5-7 lists interventions to reduce potassium levels.

Drugs and Their Effect on Potassium Balance

Potassium-wasting diuretics are a major cause of hypokalemia. Diuretics are divided into two categories: potassium-wasting and potassium-sparing drugs. Potassium-wasting diuretics excrete potassium and other electrolytes such as sodium and chloride in the urine. Potassium-sparing diuretics retain potassium but excrete sodium and chloride in the urine. Table 5-8 lists the trade and generic names of potassium-wasting and potassium-sparing diuretics and a combination of potassium-wasting and potassium-sparing diuretics.

Laxatives, corticosteroids, antibiotics, and potassium-wasting diuretics are the major drug groups that can cause hypokalemia. The drug groups attributed to hyperkalemia include oral and intravenous potassium salts, central nervous system (CNS) agents, and potassium-sparing diuretics. Table 5-9 (see page 57) lists the drugs that affect potassium balance.

Table 5-7

Correction of Potassium Excess (Hyperkalemia)

Treatment Methods	Rationale
Potassium restriction	Restriction of potassium intake will slowly lower the serum level. For mild hyperkalemia (slightly elevated K levels), i.e., 5.4–5.6 mEq/L, potassium restriction is normally effective.
IV sodium bicarbonate (NaHCO₃)	By elevating the pH level, potassium moves back into the cells, thus lowering the serum level. This is a temporary treatment.
10% Calcium gluconate	Calcium decreases the irritability of the myocardium resulting from hyperkalemia. It is a temporary treatment and does not promote K loss. *Caution:* Administering calcium to a patient on digitalis can cause digitalis toxicity.
Insulin and glucose (10–50%)	The combination of insulin and glucose moves potassium back into the cells. It is a temporary treatment, effective for approximately 6 hours, and is not always as effective when repeated.
Kayexalate (sodium polystyrene) and sorbitol 70%	Kayexalate is used as a cation exchange for severe hyperkalemia and can be administered orally or rectally. Approximate dosages are as follows: *Orally:* Kayexalate—10–20 g 3 to 4 times daily Sorbitol 70%—20 mL with each dose *Rectally:* Kayexalate—30–50 g Sorbitol 70%—50 mL; mix with 100–150 mL water (Retention enema—20–30 minutes)

● Clinical Considerations: Potassium

1. Oral potassium should be taken with food and/or 8 ounces of fluid. Potassium is irritating to the gastric mucosa and can cause a gastric ulcer.

2. Mild hypokalemia, 3.4 mEq/L, can be avoided by eating foods rich in potassium, i.e., fresh fruits, dry fruits, fruit juices, vegetables, meats, nuts.

3. Intravenous potassium should be well diluted in IV solution. NEVER administer IV potassium as a bolus (IV push). It can cause cardiac arrest.

Table 5-8

Potassium-Wasting and Potassium-Sparing Diuretics

Potassium-Wasting Diuretics	Potassium-Sparing Diuretics
Thiazides	Aldosterone antagonist
Chlorothiazide/Diuril	Spironolactone/Aldactone
Hydrochlorothiazide/Hydrodiuril	Triamterene/Dyrenium
Loop diuretics	Amiloride/Midamor
Furosemide/Lasix	
Ethacrynic acid/Edecrin	*Combination: K-Wasting and*
Carbonic anhydrase inhibitors	*K-Sparing Diuretics*
Acetazolamide/Diamox	Aldactazide
Osmotic diuretic	Spironazide
Mannitol	Dyazide
	Moduretic

4. The normal dose for IV potassium is 20–40 mEq in a liter of IV fluids to run for 8 hours.

5. Infiltration of IV potassium salt in solution causes sloughing of the subcutaneous tissues. IV potassium is irritating to blood vessels, and with prolonged use, phlebitis might occur.

6. Potassium should NOT be administered if the urine output is below 400 mL/day. Eighty to 90% of potassium is excreted in the urine.

7. Potassium deficit can enhance the action of digoxin; digitalis toxicity could result.

8. Potassium-wasting diuretics, i.e., thiazides [hydrochlorothiazide (HydroDIURIL)], and loop/high ceiling [furosemide (Lasix)] cause potassium loss via kidneys. Steroids promote potassium loss and sodium retention.

▶ CLIENT MANAGEMENT

Assessment

- Obtain a health history for clinical health problems that may cause hypokalemia or hyperkalemia.

- Assess for signs and symptoms of hypokalemia and hyperkalemia. Refer to Table 5-5.

Table 5-9

Drugs Affecting Potassium Balance

Potassium Imbalance	Substances	Rationale
Hypokalemia (serum potassium deficit)	Laxatives Enemas (hyperosmolar) Corticosteroids	Laxative abuse can cause potassium depletion.
	Cortisone	Ion exchange agent.
	Prednisone	Steroids promote potassium loss and sodium retention.
	Kayexalate	Exchange potassium ion for a sodium ion.
	Licorice	Licorice action is similar to aldosterone, promoting K loss and Na retention.
	Levodopa/L-dopa Lithium	Increases potassium loss via urine.
	Antibiotic I Amphotericin B Polymyxin B Tetracycline (outdated) Gentamicin Neomycin Amikacin Tobramycin Cisplatin	Toxic effect on renal tubules, thus decreasing potassium reabsorption.
	Antibiotic II Penicillin Ampicillin Carbenicillin Ticarcillin Nafcillin Piperacillin Azlocillin	Potassium excretion is enhanced by the presence of nonreabsorbable anions.
	Alpha-adrenergic blockers Insulin and glucose	These agents promote movement of potassium into cells, thus lowering the serum potassium level.
	Beta$_2$ agonists Terbutaline Albuterol Estrogen Potassium-wasting diuretics	See Table 5-8

continues on the following page

Table 5-9

(Continued)

Potassium Imbalance	Substances	Rationale
Hyperkalemia (serum potassium excess)	Potassium chloride (oral or IV) Potassium salt (no salt) K penicillin KPO_4 enema	Excess ingestion or infusion of these agents can cause a potassium excess.
	Indomethacin Captopril (Capoten) Heparin	Decrease renal excretion of potassium.
	CNS agents Barbiturates Sedatives Narcotics Heroin Amphetamines	These CNS agents are usually characterized by muscle necrosis and cellular shift of potassium from cells to serum.
	Nonsteroidal anti- inflammatory drugs (NSAIDS): ibuprofens Alpha agonists Beta blockers	Blocks cellular potassium uptake.
	Succinylcholine Cyclophosphamide	Loss of potassium from cells.
	Potassium-sparing diuretics	See Table 5-8.

- Check the serum potassium level that can be used as a baseline for comparison of future serum potassium levels. Recognize that a serum potassium value below 2.5 mEq/L may cause cardiac arrest.
- Check ECG strips for changes that denote hypokalemia or hyperkalemia.
- Assess vital signs and urine output. Report abnormal findings.
- Assess for signs and symptoms of digitalis toxicity, i.e., nausea, vomiting, anorexia, bradycardia, and dysrhythmias when a client is receiving a potassium-wasting diuretic and/or steroids with digoxin. Hypokalemia enhances the action of digoxin.

Diagnoses

- *Altered Nutrition, less than body requirements,* related to insufficient intake of foods rich in potassium or potassium losses (gastric suctioning)

- *Risk for Injury, Vessels, Tissues, or Gastric Mucosa,* related to phlebitis from concentrated potassium solution, infiltration of potassium solution into subcutaneous tissues, or ingestion of concentrated oral potassium irritating and damaging to the gastric mucosa

- *Risk for Cardiac Output Decreased,* related to dysrhythmia secondary to hyperkalemia

- *Altered Urinary Elimination,* related to renal dysfunction, cardiac insufficiency

Interventions

Hypokalemia

- Monitor vital signs and ECG findings.

- Monitor serum potassium values. Report serum potassium levels below 3.5 mEq/L.

- Dilute oral potassium supplements in at least 6–8 ounces of water or juice. Concentrated potassium is irritating to the gastric mucosa.

- Check infusion site for phlebitis or infiltration when KCl is administered intravenously. NEVER administer potassium intravenously as a bolus or IV push.

- Instruct clients to eat foods rich in potassium when hypokalemia is present or when the client is taking potassium-wasting diuretics and steroids. Examples of foods rich in potassium include fresh fruits, fruit juices, dry fruits, vegetables, meats, nuts, cocoa, and cola.

- Recognize other drugs and substances that decrease serum potassium levels, i.e., glucose, insulin, laxatives, licorice, lithium carbonate, salicylates, and tetracycline.

- Monitor serum magnesium, chloride, and protein when hypokalemia is present. Attempts to correct the potassium deficit may not be effective when hypomagnesemia, hypochloremia, and hypoproteinemia are present.

Hyperkalemia

- Monitor vital signs and ECG strips. Report abnormal results. Presence of peaked T wave, wide QRS complex, and prolonged P-R interval are indicative of hyperkalemia.

- Monitor serum potassium levels. Report values greater than 5.3 mEq/L.

- Monitor daily urine output. Report urine output that is less than 250 mL per 8 hours.

- Regulate IV flow rate with solution containing potassium so that no more than 10 mEq of KCl is administered per hour.

- Administer fresh blood (blood transfusion) to clients with hyperkalemia. When blood is 2–3 weeks old, the serum potassium of that blood can be very high and thus increase the risk of severe hyperkalemia.

- Monitor medical treatments for hyperkalemia. Know which corrective treatments are used for mild, moderate, and severe hyperkalemia.

Evaluation/Outcome

- Evaluate that the cause of potassium imbalance has been corrected.

- Evaluate the effect of the therapeutic regimen in correcting potassium imbalance; serum potassium levels within normal range.

- Remain free of signs and symptoms of hypokalemia or hyperkalemia; ECG, vital signs, and muscular tone are normal in pattern, range, and tone.

- Diet includes foods rich in potassium while the client is taking drugs that promote potassium loss.

- Urine output is adequate: >600 mL/day.

- Document compliance with the prescribed drug therapy and medical and dietary regimen.

Sodium and Chloride Imbalances

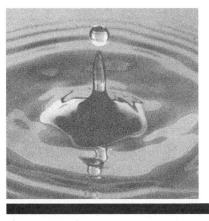

▶ INTRODUCTION

Sodium (Na) and chloride (Cl) are the principal cation and anion in the extracellular fluid (ECF). Sodium and chloride levels in the body are regulated by the kidneys and are influenced by the hormone aldosterone. Sodium is mainly responsible for water retention and the serum osmolality level. The chloride ion frequently appears in combination with the sodium ion.

The normal concentration of sodium in the extracellular fluid is 135–146 mEq/L. The normal serum chloride range is 95–108 mEq/L. A decreased serum sodium level is known as sodium deficit or **hyponatremia,** and an elevated serum sodium level is known as sodium excess or **hypernatremia.** A decreased serum chloride level is called a chloride deficit or **hypochloremia,** and an elevated serum chloride level is known as chloride excess or **hyperchloremia.** Table 6-1 includes the basic information related to sodium and chloride.

Table 6-1

Basic Information Related to Sodium and Chloride Balance

Categories	Sodium and Chloride Data
Distribution	Sodium concentration is in the extracellular fluid (ECF). Bones contain 800–1000 mEq of sodium, but only a portion of sodium is available for exchange in other parts of the body. Chloride concentration is greater in the ECF.
Functions	Sodium is important in neuromuscular activity and sodium-potassium pump action. Sodium and chloride are largely responsible for the osmolality of vascular fluids and in regulating acid-base balance. Chloride is partly responsible for the acidity in gastric juices.
Normal serum values	Sodium range is 135–146 mEq/L or 135–146 mmol/L; chloride range is 95–108 mEq/L or 95–108 mmol/L.
Normal urine value	Sodium: 40–220 mEq/L daily.
Dietary requirement	Sodium: 2–4 grams daily. Chloride: 3–9 grams daily.
Food sources	Sodium in high concentration: bacon, corned beef, ham, catsup, potato chips, pretzels with salt, pickles, olives, soda crackers, tomato juice, beef cube, dill, decaffeinated coffee. Chloride in high concentration: cheese, milk, crab, fish, dates.
Excretion	Sodium and chloride are primarily excreted via kidneys. Other avenues in excretion of Na and Cl are GI secretions and sweat.

The two most important functions of sodium are water balance and neuromuscular activity. Table 6-2 explains the multiple functions of sodium, including the sodium pump action, which is also known as the sodium-potassium pump action. The functions of chloride are given in Table 6-3. The chloride ion is an important factor in acid-base balance and the acidity of gastric juice. Chloride, like sodium, changes the serum osmolality.

▶ PATHOPHYSIOLOGY

Hyponatremia frequently occurs because of:

1. Sodium loss through the skin, GI tract, or kidneys

2. An increased amount of sodium shift into cells when there is a cellular potassium deficit

3. An excessive ADH release (SIADH) causing water retention and sodium dilution

Table 6-2

Sodium and Its Functions

Body Involvement	Functions
Neuromuscular	Transmission and conduction of nerve impulses (sodium pump—see Cellular).
Body fluids	Largely responsible for the osmolality of vascular fluids. Doubling Na level gives the approximate serum osmolality.
	Regulation of body fluid (increased sodium levels cause water retention).
Cellular	Sodium pump action. Sodium shifts into cells as potassium shifts out of the cells, repeatedly, to maintain water balance and neuromuscular activity. When Na shifts into the cell, depolarization occurs (cell activity); and when Na shifts out of the cell, K shifts back into the cell, and repolarization occurs.
	Enzyme activity.
Acid-base levels	Assist with the regulation of acid-base balance. Sodium combines readily with chloride (Cl) or bicarbonate (HCO_3) to regulate the acid-base balance.

Table 6-3

Chloride and Its Functions

Body Involvement	Functions
Osmolality (tonicity) of ECF	Chloride, like sodium, changes the serum osmolality. When serum osmolality is increased, >295 mOsm/kg, there are more sodium and chloride ions in proportion to the water. A decreased serum osmolality, <280 mOsm/kg, results in less sodium and chloride ions, and a lower serum osmolality.
Body water balance	When sodium is retained, chloride is frequently retained, causing an increase in water retention.
Acid-base balance	The kidneys excrete the anion chloride or bicarbonate, and sodium reabsorbs either chloride or bicarbonate to maintain the acid-base balance.
Acidity of gastric juice	Chloride combines with the hydrogen ion in the stomach to form hydrochloric acid (HCl).

Table 6-4

Pathophysiology of Sodium and Chloride Imbalances

Sodium Imbalances	Explanation
Hyponatremia	
Central nervous system (CNS)	The CNS is most sensitive to a decrease in the sodium level. Excess water moves into the cerebral tissues, which can result in increased intracranial pressure.
Gastrointestinal tract	Loss of sodium and chloride from the GI tract can cause acid-base imbalances.
Kidneys	Renal dysfunction promotes sodium and water retention, resulting in a diluted sodium level.
Cellular activity	A sodium deficit decreases the sodium pump action; thus, there is a decrease in cellular activity.
Hypernatremia	
Overproduction of adrenal hormones	Excess secretions of aldosterone and cortisol promote an increase in the sodium level.
Cellular activity	A sodium excess increases the sodium pump action, which can increase cellular irritability. As the hypernatremic state intensifies, less sodium passes across the cell membrane; thus, less cellular activity occurs.

Hypernatremia can occur because of:

1. Excess secretion of aldosterone or cortisol
2. Excess sodium intake

Table 6-4 describes the pathophysiology related to hyponatremia and hypernatremia.

▶ ETIOLOGY

The general causes of hyponatremia and hypochloremia are gastrointestinal losses, altered cellular function, renal losses, electrolyte-free fluids, and hormonal influences. Metabolic alkalosis can occur with hypochloremia. Table 6-5 lists the various causes and gives the rationale concerning sodium and chloride losses.

In hypernatremia and hyperchloremia, the general causes include dietary changes such as increased sodium intake with a decreased water intake, gastrointestinal disorders, decreased renal function, environmental changes, hormonal influence (excess adrenocortical hormone

Table 6-5

Causes of Hyponatremia and Hypochloremia (Serum Sodium and Chloride Deficit)

Etiology	Rationale
Dietary Changes Low-sodium diet Excessive plain water intake "Fad" diets/fasting Anorexia nervosa Prolonged use of IV D_5W	A low-sodium intake over several months can lead to hyponatremia. Drinking large quantities of plain water dilutes the ECF. Administration of continuous IV D_5W dilutes the ECF and can cause water intoxication. Gastric juice is composed of the acid hydrogen chloride (HCl).
Gastrointestinal Losses Vomiting, diarrhea GI suctioning Tap-water enemas GI surgery Bulimia Loss of potassium	Sodium and chloride are in high concentration in the gastric and intestinal mucosas. Sodium and chloride losses occur with vomiting, diarrhea, GI suctioning, and GI surgery. Loss of potassium is accompanied by loss of chloride.
Renal Losses Salt-wasting kidney disease Diuretics	In advanced renal disorders, the tubules do not respond to ADH; therefore, there is a loss of sodium, chloride, and water. The extensive use of diuretics or excessively potent diuretics can decrease the serum sodium and chloride levels.
Hormonal Influences Antidiuretic hormone (ADH), syndrome of inappropriate ADH (SIADH)	ADH promotes water reabsorption from the distal renal tubules. Surgical pain, increased use of narcotics, and head trauma cause more water to be reabsorbed, thus diluting the ECF.
Decreased adrenocortical hormone: Addison's disease	Decreased adrenocortical hormone production related to de/creased adrenal gland activity (Addison's disease) causes sodium loss and potassium retention.
Altered Cellular Function Hypervolemic state: CHF, cirrhosis	In hypervolemic states due to CHF, cirrhosis, and nephrosis, the ECF is increased, thus diluting the serum sodium and chloride levels.
Burns	Great quantities of sodium and chloride are lost from burn wounds and from oozing burn surface areas.
Skin	Large amounts of sodium and chloride are lost from the skin due to increased environmental temperature, fever, and large skin wounds.

continues on the following page.

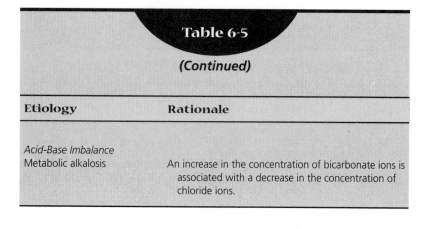

Etiology	Rationale
Acid-Base Imbalance Metabolic alkalosis	An increase in the concentration of bicarbonate ions is associated with a decrease in the concentration of chloride ions.

production), and altered cellular function. With hyperchloremia, metabolic acidosis can occur. Table 6-6 lists the causes and gives the rationale for sodium and chloride excesses.

A 24-hour urine sodium test is helpful in determining sodium retention or loss. The normal range for a 24-hour urine sodium is 40–220 mEq/L. If a client's 24-hour urine sodium is 32 mEq/L, the serum sodium level is 133 mEq/L, and the client has symptoms of heart failure, the likely cause is sodium retention.

When the client experiences severe vomiting without water replacement, the client is at risk for a sodium excess. Persistent vomiting and/or gastric suction can cause a loss of hydrogen and chloride ions; hypochloremic alkalosis can result.

▶ CLINICAL MANIFESTATIONS

The severity of clinical manifestations of hypo-hypernatremia varies with the onset and extent of sodium deficit or excess. Mild hypernatremia is normally asymptomatic, and early nonspecific symptoms such as nausea and vomiting may be overlooked. Table 6-7 gives the signs and symptoms associated with hypo-hypernatremia. Clinical manifestations of chloride imbalances are given in Table 6-8. Hypochloremic symptoms are similar to metabolic alkalosis, and hyperchloremic symptoms are similar to metabolic acidosis.

▶ CLINICAL MANAGEMENT

The majority of Americans consume 3–5 grams of sodium per day; some consume 8–15 grams daily. The daily sodium requirements are 2–4 grams. A teaspoon of salt has 2.3 grams of sodium. When sodium

Table 6-6

Causes of Hypernatremia and Hyperchloremia (Serum Sodium and Chloride Excess)

Etiology	Rationale
Dietary Changes Increased sodium intake Decreased water intake Administration of 3% saline solutions	Inadequate fluid intake and increased use of table salt, canned vegetables, and soups can increase the serum sodium and chloride levels. Administration of concentrated 3% saline solutions can cause hypernatremia and hyperchloremia.
GI Disorders Vomiting (severe) Diarrhea	With severe vomiting, water loss can be greater than sodium loss, causing a dangerously high serum sodium level. This is particularly true in babies who have diarrhea. Their loss of water can be greater than their loss of sodium.
Decreased renal function	Reduced glomerular filtration causes an excess of sodium in the body.
Environmental Changes Increased temperature and humidity Water loss	Increased environmental and body temperatures may cause profuse perspiration. Water loss can be greater than sodium and chloride losses.
Hormonal Influence Increased adrenocortical hormone production: oral or IV cortisone	Excess adrenocortical hormone can cause a sodium and chloride excess in the body whether it is due to cortisone ingestion or hyperfunction of the adrenal gland (Cushing's syndrome).
Altered Cellular Function CHF, renal diseases	Usually with CHF and renal disease, the body's sodium and chloride are greatly increased. If water retention is greatly enhanced, pseudohyponatremia may result.
Trauma: head injury	Chloride ions are frequently retained with the sodium.
Acid-base imbalance: metabolic acidosis	Increased chloride (Cl) ion concentration is associated with a decreased bicarbonate ion concentration.

Table 6-7

Clinical Manifestations of Sodium Imbalances

Body Involvement	Hyponatremia	Hypernatremia
Gastrointestinal Abnormalities	*Nausea, vomiting, diarrhea, abdominal cramps	*Nausea, vomiting, anorexia *Rough, dry tongue
Cardiac Abnormalities	Tachycardia, hypotension	*Tachycardia, possible hypertension
Central Nervous System (CNS)	*Headaches, apprehension, lethargy, confusion, depression, seizures	*Restlessness, agitation, stupor, elevated body temperature
Neuromuscular Abnormalities	*Muscular weakness	Muscular twitching, tremor, hyperreflexia
Integumentary Changes	Dry skin, pale, dry mucous membrane	*Flushed, dry skin, dry, sticky membrane
Laboratory Values		
Serum sodium	<135 mEq/L	>146 mEq/L
Urine sodium		<40 mEq/L
Specific gravity	<1.008	>1.025
Serum osmolality	<280 mOsm/kg	>295 mOsm/kg

Note: *Most common clinical manifestations of hyponatremia and hypernatremia.

Table 6-8

Clinical Manifestations of Chloride Imbalances

Body Involvement	Hypochloremia	Hyperchloremia
Neuromuscular Abnormalities	Hyperexcitability of the nerves and muscles (tremors, twitching)	Weakness Lethargy Unconsciousness (later)
Respiratory Abnormalities	Slow and shallow breathing	Deep, rapid, vigorous breathing
Cardiac Abnormalities	↓ Blood pressure with severe Cl and ECF losses	
Laboratory Values		
Milliequivalent per liter	<95 mEq/L	>108 mEq/L

intake increases, the water intake also tends to increase. As a result of the sodium and water increase, extracellular fluid is increased.

When the serum sodium level is <130 mEq/L (hyponatremia), a saline solution to restore sodium balance is usually administered. The suggested sodium replacement includes:

> **Sodium Replacement According to the Serum Sodium Level**
> Serum sodium: <130 mEq/L = normal saline solution
> (0.9% NaCl)
> Serum sodium: <115 mEq/L = 3% saline solution

When giving 3% saline solution, the client should be closely monitored for a fluid overload and pulmonary edema.

To correct hypernatremia, the cause should be known and corrected. If the client is consuming an excess amount of salt, then salt restriction should be enforced. If the cause of hypernatremia is congestive heart failure (CHF), medical treatment should be prescribed.

Drugs and Their Effect on Sodium Balance

The drug categories of certain antidepressant groups, certain anticancer drugs, oral antidiabetics, and certain CNS depressants (morphine, barbiturates) can cause hyponatremia. Corticosteroids, certain antibiotics, and ingestion and infusion of sodium are causes of hypernatremia. Table 6-9 lists the drugs that affect sodium balance.

● Clinical Considerations: Sodium and Chloride

1. Serum osmolality of body fluids (ECF) can be estimated by *doubling the serum sodium level.* For a more accurate serum osmolality level, use the formula

$$2 \times \text{serum Na} + \frac{\text{BUN}}{3} + \frac{\text{glucose}}{18} = \frac{\text{serum osmolality}}{\text{(mOsm/kg)}}$$

The normal serum osmolality range is 280–295 mOsm/kg.

2. Sodium causes water retention.

3. One teaspoon of salt is equivalent to 2.3 grams of sodium. Daily sodium requirement is 2–4 grams. Most Americans consume 3–5 grams of sodium per day, and some consume 8–15 grams daily.

Table 6-9

Drugs Affecting Sodium Balance

Sodium Imbalance	Drugs	Rationale
Hyponatremia (serum sodium deficit)	Diuretics	Diuretics, either K- wasting or K-sparing, cause sodium excretion.
	Lithium	Lithium promotes urinary sodium loss.
	Antineoplastics/Anticancer Vincristine Cyclophosphamide Cisplatin Antipsychotics Amitryptyline (Elavil) Thioridazine (Mellaril) Thiothixene (Navane) Tranylcypromine (Parnate) Antidiabetics Chlorpropamide (Diabenase) Tolbutamide (Orinase) CNS depressants Morphine Barbiturates Ibuprofens (Motrin) Nicotine Clonidine (Catapres)	Anticancer drugs, antipsychotics, and antidiabetics stimulate ADH release and cause hemodilution and decrease sodium level.
Hypernatremia (serum sodium excess)	Corticosteroids Cortisone Prednisone	Steroids promote sodium retention and potassium excretion.
	Hypertonic saline Sodium salicylate Sodium phosphate Sodium bicarbonate Cough medicines	Administration of sodium salts in excess.
	Antibiotics Azlocillin Na Penicillin Na	Many of the antibiotics contain the sodium salt, which increases drug absorption.
	Mezlocillin Na Carbenicillin Ticarcillin disodium	Ion exchange.

continues on the following page

Table 6-9

(Continued)

Sodium Imbalance	Drugs	Rationale
Hypernatremia (serum sodium excess) (cont'd)	Cholestyramine Amphotericin B Demeclocycline Propoxyphene (Darvon)	These miscellaneous drugs promote urinary water loss without sodium.
	Lactulose	Water loss in excess of sodium via GI tract.

4. Vomiting causes sodium and chloride losses, and diarrhea causes sodium, chloride, and bicarbonate losses.

5. A 3% saline solution should be given when there is a severe serum sodium deficit, e.g., <115 mEq/L. When administering a 3% saline solution, check for signs and symptoms of pulmonary edema.

6. A serum potassium cannot be fully corrected until the chloride deficit is corrected.

7. Sodium and potassium have opposite effects on cellular activity. The sodium pump effect causes sodium to shift into the cells, resulting in depolarization. When sodium shifts out of the cells, potassium shifts into cells and repolarization occurs. The sodium pump action is continuously repeated.

8. Continuous use of a saline solution causes a calcium loss.

9. Steroids promote sodium retention and, thus, water retention. Cough medicine, sulfonamides, and some antibiotics containing sodium can increase the serum sodium level.

▶ CLIENT MANAGEMENT

Assessment

• Obtain a history of high-risk factors for decreased and increased serum sodium and chloride levels. Examples of hyponatremia include GI losses, eating disorders such as anorexia nervosa and bulimia, continuous use of 5% dextrose in water, and potent diuretics. Examples of hypernatremia include increased salt intake, renal and cardiac diseases, and increased production of aldosterone.

- Assess for signs and symptoms of hyponatremia or hypernatremia.

- Obtain serum sodium and chloride levels that can be used as baseline values for future comparison.

- Check the serum osmolality level. A serum osmolality value of <280 mOsm/kg indicates hyponatremia and a serum osmolality of >295 mOsm/kg indicates hypernatremia.

Diagnoses

- *Altered Electrolyte, Sodium,* related to vomiting, diarrhea, gastric suction, SIADH resulting from surgery, potent diuretics

- *Altered Nutrition, more than body requirements,* related to excess intake of foods rich in sodium

- *Impaired Skin Integrity,* related to peripheral edema secondary to sodium and water excess

Interventions

Hyponatremia

- Monitor the serum sodium and chloride levels. Sodium replacement with chloride may be needed if the serum sodium deficit is due to GI losses. Hypervolemic conditions such as CHF can indicate pseudo-hyponatremia.

- Keep an accurate intake and output record. Excess water intake can cause hyponatremia and hypochloremia related to hemodilution.

- Observe changes in vital signs, i.e., pulse rate. Shocklike symptoms can occur if hyponatremia is due to hypovolemia.

- Restrict water when hyponatremia is due to hypervolemia.

- Administer a 3% saline solution (for severe sodium deficit) cautiously. Check for signs of fluid overload and pulmonary edema.

Hypernatremia

- Instruct the client with hypernatremia to avoid foods rich in salt, i.e., canned foods, lunch meats, ham, pickles, and salted potato chips and pretzels.

- Monitor the serum sodium level. Check for chest rales and for edema in the lower extremities.

- Identify drugs the client is taking that could have a sodium-retaining effect, such as cortisone preparations, cough medicines, and certain laxatives containing sodium.

Hypochloremia and Hyperchloremia

- Monitor arterial blood gases when an acid-base imbalance is suspected. With hypochloremia, metabolic alkalosis can result, and with hyperchloremia, metabolic acidosis can occur.

Evaluation/Outcome

- Evaluate that the cause of sodium and chloride imbalances has been corrected or controlled.

- Evaluate the effect of the therapeutic regimen on the correction of sodium and chloride imbalances; serum sodium and chloride levels should be periodically checked.

- Remain free of signs and symptoms of hyponatremia and hypernatremia.

- Check that fluid imbalances are not contributing to sodium and chloride imbalances; the client is not dehydrated or overhydrated.

- Determine that the urine output has been adequate, >600 mL/day.

Calcium Imbalances

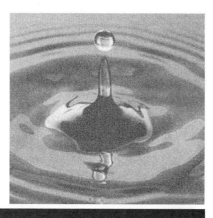

▶ INTRODUCTION

Calcium (Ca) is found in both the extracellular and intracellular fluids; however, it is somewhat more concentrated in the extracellular fluid. Approximately 55% of serum calcium is bound to protein and 45% is free ionized calcium. It is the free calcium that is physiologically active.

The serum calcium concentration range is 4.5–5.5 mEq/L, 9–11 mg/dL, or 2.23–2.57 mmol/L. A decrease in the serum calcium level is known as **hypocalcemia,** and an increase in serum calcium level is called **hypercalcemia.** Today's blood analyzers allow the ionized calcium (iCa) level to be measured. The normal serum ionized calcium range is 2.2–2.5 mEq/L, 4.25–5.25 mg/dL, or 1.15–1.30 mmol/L. Certain changes in the blood composition can either increase or decrease the serum iCa level. When an individual is acidotic, calcium is released from the serum protein and increases the serum iCa level. During alkalosis, calcium is bound to protein and there is less iCa.

Vitamin D is needed for calcium absorption from the gastrointestinal tract. The anion phosphorus (P) inhibits calcium absorption. Thus, the

Table 7-1

Basic Information Related to Calcium Balance

Categories	Calcium Data
Distribution	Ninety-nine percent of calcium is in teeth and bones; 1% is in the extracellular fluid (ECF) and intracellular fluid (ICF), with the greater concentration of the 1% in the ECF.
Functions	Includes neuromuscular activity, maintaining cardiac contraction and cellular permeability, promoting blood clotting and the formation of teeth and bone.
Normal serum values	Calcium (Ca): 4.5–5.5 mEq/L, 9–11 mg/dL Ionized calcium (iCa): 2.2–2.5 mEq/L, 4.25–5.25 mg/dL
Normal excretion (urine)	Two hundred milligrams per day.
Dietary requirement	Eight hundred milligrams daily.
Food sources	Milk, cheese, vegetables (baked beans, kale, greens, broccoli), meats, salmon.
Excretion	Urine: 200 mg/day; bile: 200 mg/day; others: pancreatic and intestinal (feces) secretions.

actions of these two ions on the body have an opposite physiologic effect. Both calcium and phosphorus are stored in the bones and excreted by the kidneys. Table 7-1 includes the basic information regarding calcium balance.

The parathyroid glands secrete the parathyroid hormone (PTH), which is responsible for the homeostatic regulation of the calcium ion in body fluids. The parathyroid glands are located on the posterior thyroid gland. When the serum calcium level is low, the parathyroid glands secrete more parathyroid hormone (PTH); PTH increases the calcium level by promoting calcium release from the bone as needed. Calcitonin from the thyroid gland increases calcium return to the bone, decreasing the serum calcium level. Figure 7-1 diagrams the sequence and actions of PTH and calcitonin from the parathyroid and thyroid glands on the bone.

Calcium is needed for neuromuscular activity, contraction of the myocardium, normal cellular permeability, coagulation of blood, and bone and teeth formation. Table 7-2 explains the functions of calcium.

▶ PATHOPHYSIOLOGY

A serum calcium level less than 4.5 mEq/L, or 9mg/dL, is known as hypocalcemia and a serum calcium level greater than 5.5 mEq/L, or 11mg/dL, is known as hypercalcemia. Muscles (skeletal, smooth, and cardiac) and

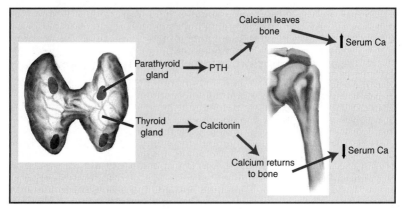

Figure 7-1 Functions of PTH and Calcitonin

Table 7-2

Calcium and Its Functions

Body Involvement	Functions
Neuromuscular	Normal nerve and muscle activity. Calcium causes transmission of nerve impulses and contraction of skeletal muscles.
Cardiac	Contraction of heart muscle (myocardium).
Cellular and Blood	Maintenance of normal cellular permeability. ↑ calcium decreases cellular permeability and ↓ calcium increases cellular permeability. Coagulation of blood. Calcium promotes blood clotting by converting prothrombin into thrombin.
Bones and Teeth	Formation of bone and teeth. Calcium and phosphorus make bones and teeth strong and durable.

nerves (peripheral) are affected by hypocalcemia. Table 7-3 explains the pathophysiologic effects of calcium imbalances.

▶ ETIOLOGY

The causes of hypocalcemia include dietary changes, renal dysfunction, hormonal and electrolyte influences, and multiple citrated blood transfusions. Table 7-4 lists these causes and the rationale. Lack of calcium intake, inadequate vitamin D, and lack of protein in the diet are some major causes of hypocalcemia.

Table 7-3

Pathophysiology of Calcium Imbalances

Calcium Imbalance	Explanations
Hypocalcemia	
Parathyroid hormone (PTH)	Decreased PTH level causes calcium release from bones to be inhibited.
Neuromuscular	Excitability of the skeletal, smooth, and cardiac muscles.
Bone	A prolonged serum calcium deficit leads to osteoporosis.
Clotting time	A marked serum calcium deficit impairs the clotting time and clot formation. A decrease in blood coagulation results in bleeding.
Electrolyte: magnesium	A severe magnesium deficit results in a calcium deficit. PTH secretions are decreased when there is a magnesium deficit; thus, the serum calcium level is decreased.
Hypercalcemia	
Gastrointestinal	Hypercalcemia decreases GI peristalsis and GI motility. An increased calcium level enhances hydrochloric acid, gastrin, and pancreatic enzyme release.
Cardiac	A calcium excess decreases cardiac activity. Dysrhythmias, heart block, and ECG/EKG changes can occur.
Altered cellular changes	Hypercalcemia decreases cellular permeability.
Bones	A calcium excess frequently results in calcium loss from the bones. An elevated serum calcium level usually results from bone loss because of malignancy or prolonged immobilization.

The causes of hypercalcemia include dietary changes, renal impairment, cellular destruction, and hormonal and drug influence. Table 7-5 lists these causes and the rationale. The thiazide diuretics promote calcium retention; however, the loop diuretics cause calcium loss.

▶ CLINICAL MANIFESTATIONS

Signs of hypocalcemia and hypercalcemia are ECG/EKG changes, the serum calcium level, and the serum ionized calcium level. A commonly seen clinical manifestation of hypocalcemia is tetany. Positive Chvostek's and Trousseau's signs indicate hypocalcemia. Figure 7-2 (see page 80) describes the

Table 7-4

Causes of Hypocalcemia (Serum Calcium Deficit)

Etiology	Rationale
Dietary Changes	
Lack of calcium intake, inadequate vitamin D, and/or lack of protein in diet	A calcium (Ca) deficit resulting from lack of Ca intake is rare. Vitamin D must be present for calcium absorption from GI tract. Inadequate protein intake inhibits the body's utilization of calcium.
Chronic diarrhea	Chronic diarrhea interferes with adequate calcium absorption.
Renal Dysfunction	
Renal failure	Renal failure causes phosphorus and calcium retention. Lack of PTH decreases renal calcium absorption.
Hormonal and Electrolyte Influence	
Decreased parathyroid hormone (PTH) Increased serum phosphorus (phosphate) Increased serum magnesium Severe decreased magnesium Increased calcitonin	With hypoparathyroidism, there is less PTH secreted. Secondary hypoparathyroidism may be caused by sepsis, burns, surgery, or pancreatitis. Overuse of phosphate laxatives can decrease calcium retention. Magnesium imbalances inhibit PTH secretion.
Calcium Binders or Chelators	
Citrated blood transfusions	Rapid administration of citrated blood binds with calcium, inhibiting ionized (free) Ca.
Alkalosis	Alkalosis increases calcium protein binding.
Increased serum albumin level	With an increase in serum albumin, more calcium is bound and less calcium is free and active.

technique for checking Chvostek's and Trousseau's signs. Table 7-6 (see page 81) lists the clinical manifestations for hypocalcemia and hypercalcemia.

Figure 7-3 (see page 82) displays two ECG strips that reflect the ECG/EKG changes resulting from either hypocalcemia or hypercalcemia.

Table 7-5

Causes of Hypercalcemia (Serum Calcium Excess)

Etiology	Rationale
Dietary Changes: Increased Calcium Salts (supplements)	Excessive use of calcium supplements, calcium salts, and antacids can increase the serum calcium level.
Renal Impairment, Diuretics: Thiazides	Kidney dysfunction and use of thiazide diuretics decrease the excretion of calcium.
Cellular Destruction Bone Immobility	A malignant bone tumor, a fracture, and/or a prolonged immobilization can cause loss of calcium from the bone. Some malignancies cause an ectopic PTH production. Increased immobility promotes calcium loss from the bone.
Hormonal and Drug Influence Increased PTH	Hyperparathyroidism increases the production of PTH and increased PTH, then promotes the release of calcium from the bone.
Decreased serum phosphorus	A decreased phosphorus level can increase the serum calcium level to the extent that the kidneys are unable to excrete excess calcium.
Steroid therapy	Steroids such as cortisone mobilize calcium absorption from the bone.
Thiazide diuretics	Thiazides increase the action of PTH on kidneys, promoting calcium reabsorption.

▶ CLINICAL MANAGEMENT

Clinical management of hypocalcemia consists of oral supplements and intravenous calcium diluted in 5% dextrose in water (D_5W). Calcium should NOT be diluted in a normal saline solution (0.9% NaCl) because the sodium encourages calcium loss. Table 7-7 (see page 83) lists the oral and intravenous preparations of calcium salts and their dosages and drug form. Calcium carbonate can cause GI upset because it produces carbon dioxide. For better calcium absorption, calcium supplements should contain vitamin D and oral calcium should be taken 30 minutes before meals.

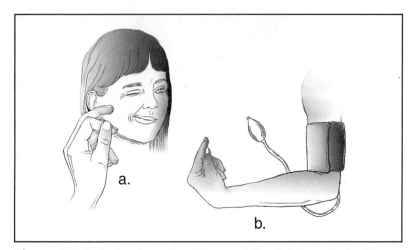

Figure 7-2 Testing for Chovstek's and Trousseau's Signs (a.) Chovstek's sign: The face is tapped over the facial nerve (2cm anterior to the earlobe). A positive test results when the facial muscle twitches. (b.) Trousseau's sign: Inflate a blood pressure cuff (20-30 mm Hg) on the upper arm to constrict circulation. A positive Trousseau is evidenced as the occurrence of a carpopedal spasm of the finger and hands within 1-5 minutes.

The goal for managing hypercalcemia is to correct the underlying cause of the serum calcium excess. Drugs such as calcitonin or IV saline solution administered rapidly and followed by a loop diuretic can be used to promote rapid urinary excretion of calcium. Table 7-8 (see page 83) gives guidelines for the suggested clinical management for hypocalcemia.

Malignancies are a common cause of hypercalcemia. A metastatic bone lesion can destroy the bone, which releases calcium into the circulation, thus elevating the serum calcium level. Some cancers promote the secretion of the parathyroid hormone (PTH) and may be referred to as tumor-secreting (ectopic) PTH production. The most common types of cancer that cause hypercalcemia are lung, breast, ovary, prostate, leukemia, and gastrointestinal cancers. The antitumor antibiotic plicamycin (mithramycin) inhibits the action of PTH on osteoclasts in the bone and decreases the serum calcium level.

Drugs and Their Effect on Calcium Balance

Phosphate preparations, corticosteroids, loop diuretics, aspirin, anticonvulsants, magnesium sulfate, and mithramycin are some of the groups of drugs that can lower the serum calcium level. Excess calcium salt ingestion and infusion and thiazide and chlorthalidone diuretics can increase the serum calcium level. Table 7-9 (see page 84) lists the drugs that affect calcium balance.

Table 7-6

Clinical Manifestations of Calcium Imbalances

Body Involvement	Hypocalcemia	Hypercalcemia

CNS and Muscular Abnormalities	Anxiety, irritability
	Tetany
	  Twitching around mouth
	  Tingling and numbness of fingers
	  Carpopedal spasm
	  Spasmodic contractions
	  Laryngeal spasm
	  Convulsions
	Abdominal cramps
	Muscle cramps
		Depression/apathy
		Muscles are flabby

Chvostek's Sign	Positive	
Trousseau's Sign	Positive	
Cardiac Abnormalities	Weak cardiac contractions	Signs of heart block Cardiac arrest in systole
ECG/EKG	Lengthened ST segment Prolonged QT interval	Decreased or diminished ST segment Shortened QT interval
Blood Abnormalities	Blood does not clot normally, reduction of prothrombin.	
Skeletal Abnormalities	Fractures occur if deficit persists.	Pathologic fractures Deep pain over bony areas Thinning of bones apparent
Renal Abnormalities		Flank pain Calcium stones formed in the kidney
Laboratory Values		
Serum Ca	<4.5 mEq/L	>5.5 mEq/L
Ionized serum Ca	<2.2 mEq/L	>2.5 mEq/L
Serum Ca	<9.0 mg/dL	>11.0 mg/dL
Ionized serum Ca	<4.25 mg/dL	>5.25 mg/dL

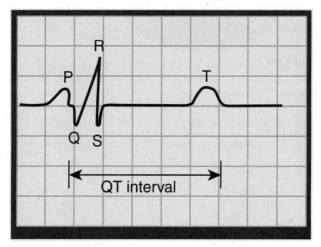

Figure 7-3A
Lengthened ST Segment
Prolonged QT Interval

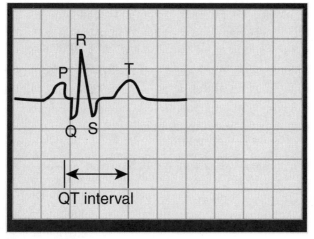

Figure 7-3B
Decreased ST Segment
Shortened QT Interval

● Clinical Considerations: Calcium

1. Administer an oral calcium supplement containing vitamin D. Vitamin D is necessary for intestinal absorption of calcium.

2. Oral calcium supplements with vitamin D should be given 30 minutes before meals to improve GI absorption.

Table 7-7

Calcium Preparations

Calcium Name	Drug Form	Drug Dose
Orals		
Calcium carbonate	650–1500 mg tablets	400 mg/g*
Calcium citrate	950-mg tablet	211 mg/g*
Calcium lactate	325–650 mg tablets	130 mg/g*
Calcium gluconate	500–1000-mg tablets	90 mg/g*
Intravenous		
Calcium chloride	10 mL size	272 mg/g*; 13.5 mEq
Calcium gluceptate	5 mL size	90 mg/g*; 4.5 mEq
Calcium gluconate	10 mL size	90 mg/g*; 4.5 mEq

*Elemental calcium is 1 gram (1g).

Table 7-8

Suggested Clinical Management for Hypocalcemia

Calcium Deficit	Suggested Clinical Management
Mild	Oral calcium salts with vitamin D, take twice a day. 10% IV calcium gluconate (10 mL) in D_5W solution. Administer slowly, 1–3 mL/min.
Moderate	10% IV calcium gluconate (10–20 mL) in D_5W solution. Administer slowly, 1–3 mL/min.
Severe	10% IV calcium gluconate (100 mL) in 1 liter of D_5W. Administer over 4 hours.

3. Intravenous calcium salts should be diluted in 5% dextrose in water (D_5W). Do NOT dilute calcium salts in a saline solution; sodium promotes calcium loss.

4. The suggested IV flow rate for a calcium solution is 1–3 mL/min (average: 2 mL/min).

5. Infiltration of calcium solution, especially calcium chloride, can cause sloughing of the subcutaneous tissues.

6. An elevated serum calcium level can enhance the action of digoxin, causing digitalis toxicity.

Table 7-9

Drugs Affecting Calcium Balance

Calcium Imbalance	Drugs	Rationale
Hypocalcemia (serum calcium deficit)	Magnesium sulfate Propylthiouracil/Propacil Colchicine Plicamycin/Mithracin Neomycin Excessive sodium citrate	These agents inhibit parathyroid hormone/PTH secretion and decrease the serum calcium level.

	Acetazolamide
	Aspirin
	Anticonvulsants
	Glutethimide/Doriden
	Estrogens
	Aminoglycosides
	  Gentamicin
	  Amikacin
	  Tobramycin
		These agents can alter the vitamin D metabolism that is needed for calcium absorption.

	Phosphate preparations:
	Oral, enema, and intravenous
	  Sodium phosphate
	  Potassium phosphate
		Phosphates can increase the serum phosphorus level and decrease the serum calcium level.

	Corticosteroids
	  Cortisone
	  Prednisone
		Steroids decrease calcium mobilization and inhibit the absorption of calcium.

	Loop diuretics Furosemide/Lasix	Loop diuretics reduce calcium absorption from the renal tubules.
Hypercalcemia (serum calcium excess)	Calcium salts Vitamin D	Excess ingestion of calcium and vitamin D and infusion of calcium can increase the serum Ca level.
	IV lipids	Lipids can increase the calcium level.

	Kayexalate, androgens
	Diuretics
	  Thiazides
	  Chlorthalidone/Hygroten
		These agents can induce hypercalcemia.

7. Diuretics such as furosemide (Lasix) can decrease the serum calcium level, and thiazide diuretics tend to increase the serum calcium levels. Steroids decrease serum calcium levels.

▶ CLIENT MANAGEMENT

Assessment

- Obtain a health history to identify potential causes of hypocalcemia or hypercalcemia; see Tables 7-4 and 7-5.

- Assess for signs and symptoms of hypocalcemia or hypercalcemia. Tetany symptoms (twitching around mouth, carpopedal spasms, laryngospasms) occur with a severe calcium deficit.

- Obtain a serum calcium level that can be used as a baseline for comparison of future serum calcium levels. A serum calcium level <4.5 mEq/L or <9 mg/dL or iCa<2.2 mEq/L indicates hypocalcemia. A serum calcium level >5.5 mEq/L or >11 mg/dL or iCa >2.5 mEq/L indicates hypercalcemia.

- Check ECG/EKG strips for changes that are indicative of a calcium imbalance.

- Determine the acid-base status when hypocalcemia is present. In an acidotic state, calcium is ionized and can be utilized by the body even though there is a calcium deficit.

- Assess for positive Trousseau's or Chvostek's signs when hypocalcemia is suspected.

- Identify drugs that the client is taking that contribute to a calcium imbalance.

Diagnoses

- *Altered Nutrition, less than body requirements,* related to insufficient calcium intake, poor calcium absorption due to insufficient vitamin D and protein intake, or drugs (antacids, cortisone preparations) that interfere with calcium ionization.

- *Risk for Injury, bleeding,* related to the interference with blood coagulation secondary to calcium loss.

- *Risk for Injury,* related to pathologic fractures due to bone destruction from bone cancer, prolonged immobilization, and hypercalcemia.

- *Altered Urinary Elimination,* related to causes of hypercalcemia.

Interventions

Hypocalcemia

- Monitor serum calcium levels, vital signs, and ECG strips for changes.
- Monitor intravenous solutions that contain calcium; infiltration can cause sloughing of the subcutaneous tissues.
- Administer oral calcium supplements at least 30 minutes prior to a meal to enhance intestinal absorption.
- Regulate IV 10% calcium gluconate or chloride in a liter of 5% dextrose in water to run 1–3 mL/min. Do not administer calcium salts in an IV normal saline solution. Sodium encourages calcium loss.
- Teach clients to eat foods rich in calcium, vitamin D, and protein, especially the older adult. Tell the client that protein is needed to aid in calcium absorption.
- Explain to persons using antacids that constant use of antacids can decrease calcium in the body. Antacids decrease acidity, thus decreasing calcium ionization.
- Check for prolonged bleeding or reduced clot formation. A low serum calcium level inhibits the production of prothrombin, which is needed in clot formation.

Hypercalcemia

- Monitor serum calcium levels, vital signs, and ECG strips, noting any changes.
- Promote active and passive exercises for bedridden clients. Immobilization promotes calcium loss from the bone.
- Identify symptoms of digitalis toxicity (bradycardia, nausea, vomiting, visual disturbances). An elevated serum calcium level while receiving a digitalis preparation enhances the action of digoxin.
- Teach the client with hypercalcemia to maintain hydration. Increased hydration increases calcium dilution and prevents renal calculi formation.
- Instruct clients with hypercalcemia to avoid foods rich in calcium.
- Monitor urinary output and urine pH. Calcium precipitates in alkaline urine and renal calculi can result. Acid-ash foods and juices such as cranberry and prune juices should be encouraged to increase the acidity of the urine. Acid urine increases the solubility of calcium. Orange juice will not change the urine pH.

- Instruct clients to increase fluid intake to dilute the serum and urine levels of calcium and to prevent the formation of renal calculi.

- Administer prescribed loop diuretics (Lasix) to enhance calcium excretion. Thiazide diuretics inhibit calcium excretion and are not indicated in hypercalcemia.

Evaluation/Outcome

- Evaluate the cause of calcium imbalance and document corrective measures taken.

- Evaluate the effects of the prescribed therapeutic regimen for hypocalcemia or hypercalcemia; serum calcium and ionized calcium levels within normal range.

- Remain free of signs and symptoms of hypocalcemia; absence of tetany symptoms, vital signs are within normal range.

- Include foods rich in calcium, such as dairy products; oral calcium supplements with vitamin D.

- Document compliance with the prescribed drug therapy and medical and dietary regimen.

Magnesium Imbalances

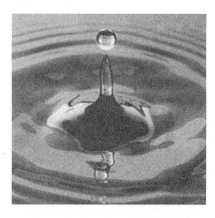

▶ INTRODUCTION

Magnesium (Mg), the second most plentiful intracellular cation, has similar functions, causes of imbalances, and clinical manifestations as potassium. The normal serum magnesium level is 1.5–2.5 mEq/L or 1.8–3.0 mg/dL. A serum magnesium deficit is known as **hypomagnesemia,** and a serum magnesium excess is called **hypermagnesemia.**

One-third of magnesium is protein bound and approximately two-thirds is ionized, free magnesium that can be utilized by the body. Magnesium is absorbed from the small intestine. Table 8-1 provides the basic information related to magnesium balance.

Magnesium plays an important role in neuromuscular, cardiac, and enzyme activities. Magnesium acts as a coenzyme in the metabolism of carbohydrates and protein. Table 8-2 summarizes the various functions of magnesium.

Table 8-1

Basic Information Related to Magnesium Balance

Categories	Magnesium Data
Distribution	Fifty percent of magnesium (Mg) is in bones; 49% of Mg is in intracellular fluid (ICF), and 1% is in extracellular fluid (ECF).
Functions	Influences neuromuscular activity, aids other electrolytes with cardiac contractions, activates many enzymes, and influences the utilization of K, Ca, and protein.
Normal serum values	Mg: 1.5– 2.5 mEq/L; 1.8–3.0 mg/dL; 0.65–1.1 mmol/L.
Normal excretion (urine)	Mg: 120–140 mg daily.
Dietary daily requirement	For adults: 300–350 mg; for infants: 150 mg.
Food sources	Green vegetables, whole grains, fish and seafood, and nuts.
Excretion	Sixty percent is excreted in feces and 40% via kidneys.

Table 8-2

Magnesium and Its Functions

Body Involvement	Functions
Neuromuscular	Transmits neuromuscular activity. Important mediator of neural transmission in the CNS.
Cardiac	Contracts the heart muscle (myocardium).
Cellular	Activates many enzymes for proper carbohydrate and protein metabolism. Responsible for the transportation of sodium and potassium across cell membranes. Influences utilization of potassium, calcium, and protein. Magnesium deficits are frequently accompanied by a potassium and/or calcium deficit.

▶ PATHOPHYSIOLOGY

Excess magnesium can cause a sedative effect on the neuromuscular system by inhibiting neuromuscular responses. A magnesium deficit increases neuromuscular excitability. Table 8-3 describes the pathophysiologic factors related to hypomagnesemia and hypermagnesemia.

▶ ETIOLOGY

Hypomagnesemia is probably the most frequently undiagnosed electrolyte deficiency. The total serum magnesium concentration is not representative of the cellular magnesium levels. Clients with hypomagnesemia are asymptomatic until the serum magnesium level approaches 1.0 mEq/L. Hence, many clients with hypomagnesemia are asymptomatic. Clients with hypokalemia or hypocalcemia who do not respond to potassium and/or calcium replacement may also have hypomagnesemia. Correction of the magnesium deficit should be seriously considered when correcting serum potassium and serum calcium imbalances.

The causes of hypomagnesemia and hypermagnesemia are presented in two tables. Table 8-4 lists the etiology and rationale for hypomagnesemia, and Table 8-5 lists the etiology and rationale for hypermagnesemia.

Table 8-3

Pathophysiology of Magnesium Imbalances

Magnesium Imbalance	Explanation
Hypomagnesemia	
Neuromuscular	Magnesium (Mg) deficit increases neuromuscular excitability. Mg deficit increases the release of acetylcholine from the presynaptic membrane of nerve fibers.
Cardiac	Can cause tachycardia, hypertension, cardiac dysrhythmias, ventricular fibrillation.
Gastrointestinal	GI dysfunction can inhibit Mg absorption from the small intestine.
Hormonal	Magnesium inhibits the release of the parathyroid hormone (PTH), which can cause a calcium deficit because of the decreased PTH.
Hypermagnesemia	
Neuromuscular	A serum Mg excess has a sedative effect on the neuromuscular system, resulting in a loss of deep tendon reflexes.
Cardiac	Hypermagnesemia can cause hypotension and heart block.
Respiratory	Can inhibit intercostal muscle action, thus decreasing respirations, which could result in respiratory paralysis.
Renal	Renal insufficiency can increase the magnesium level since 40% of magnesium is excreted by the kidneys.

Table 8-4

Causes of Hypomagnesemia (Serum Magnesium Deficit)

Etiology	Rationale
Dietary Changes	
Inadequate intake, poor absorption, GI losses	Magnesium is found in various foods, e.g., green, leafy vegetables and whole grains.
Malnutrition, starvation	Inadequate nutrition can result in a magnesium deficit.
Total parenteral nutrition (TPN, hyperalimentation)	Continuous use of TPN without a magnesium supplement can cause a magnesium deficit.
Chronic alcoholism	Alcoholism promotes inadequate food intake and GI loss of magnesium.
Increased calcium intake	Calcium absorption promotes magnesium loss in feces.
Chronic diarrhea, intestinal fistulas, chronic use of laxatives	Chronic diarrhea impairs magnesium absorption. Prolonged use of laxatives can cause a magnesium deficit.
Renal Dysfunction	
Diuresis: diabetic ketoacidosis	Diuresis due to diabetic ketoacidosis causes magnesium loss via the kidneys.
Acute renal failure (ARF)	ARF in the diuretic phase promotes magnesium loss.
Cardiac Dysfunction	
Acute myocardial infarction (AMI)	Hypomagnesemia may occur from the first to the fifth day post-acute MI.
Congestive heart failure (CHF)	Prolonged diuretic therapy for CHF can cause a magnesium deficit.
Electrolyte Influence	
Hypokalemia	The cations potassium and calcium are interrelated with magnesium action.
Hypocalcemia	Hypomagnesemia can occur with hypokalemia and hypocalcemia.
Drug Influence	
Aminoglycosides, potassium-wasting diuretics, cortisone, amphotericin B, digitalis	These drugs promote the loss of magnesium. Hypomagnesemia enhances the action of digitalis; digitalis toxicity may result.

Table 8-5

Causes of Hypermagnesemia (Serum Magnesium Excess)

Etiology	Rationale
Dietary Changes Excessive administration of magnesium products IV magnesium sulfate Antacids with magnesium Laxatives with magnesium	Hypermagnesemia rarely occurs unless there is a prolonged excess use of magnesium-containing antacids (Maalox), laxatives (milk of magnesia), and IV magnesium sulfate.
Renal Dysfunction Renal insufficiency Renal failure	Renal insufficiency or failure inhibits the excretion of magnesium.
Severe Dehydration Diabetic ketoacidosis	Loss of body fluids due to diuresis from diabetic ketoacidosis causes a hemoconcentration of magnesium, which can result in an increased magnesium level.

▶ CLINICAL MANIFESTATIONS

Magnesium influences the nervous system; too much or not enough magnesium affects the neuromuscular function. Severe hypomagnesemia may result in symptoms of tetany. Weakness, loss of deep tendon reflexes, and paralysis are signs and symptoms of hypermagnesemia. Central nervous system depression inhibits neuromuscular transmission, thus decreasing muscle tone and respiration. The serum magnesium level and the ECG changes determine the severity of the magnesium imbalance. Table 8–6 lists the clinical manifestations of hypomagnesemia and hypermagnesemia.

A **magnesium tolerance (load) test** may be prescribed to determine the presence of hypomagnesemia. With this test, a magnesium product is infused over 4–12 hours (check the procedure). Urine is collected over 24 hours starting with the beginning of the infusion. The normal magnesium excretion is 60–80% in 24 hours. Abnormal findings represent less than 50% of magnesium excretion.

Table 8-6

Clinical Manifestations of Magnesium Imbalances

Body Involvement	Hypomagnesemia	Hypermagnesemia
Neuromuscular abnormalities	Hyperirritability Tetanylike symptoms Tremors Twitching of face Spasticity Increased tendon reflexes	CNS depression Lethargy, drowsiness, weakness, paralysis Loss of deep tendon reflexes
Cardiac abnormalities	Hypertension Cardiac dysrhythmias Premature ventricular contractions Ventricular tachycardia Ventricular fibrillation	Hypotension (if severe, profound hypotension) Complete heart block
ECG/EKG	Flat or inverted T wave Depressed ST segment	Widened QRS complex Prolonged QT interval
Others		Flushing Respiratory depression

▶ CLINICAL MANAGEMENT

Clinical management of hypomagnesemia includes a diet consisting of green vegetables, legumes, nuts (peanut butter), and fruits. Oral or intravenous magnesium salts may be prescribed when there is a marked to severe magnesium deficit. Table 8–7 lists the methods of clinical management for hypomagnesemia. Correction for magnesium deficit may take 3–4 days, depending upon the severity of the deficit.

Correcting hypermagnesemia should include underlying causes and using intravenous saline or calcium salts to decrease the serum magnesium level. Intravenous calcium is an antagonist to magnesium; therefore, calcium decreases the symptoms of hypermagnesemia. If renal failure is the cause of severe hypermagnesemia, dialysis may be necessary.

Drugs and Their Effect on Magnesium Balance

Sodium inhibits tubular absorption of magnesium and calcium. Long-term administration of saline infusions may result in losses of

Table 8-7

Suggested Clinical Management for Hypomagnesemia

Drug Name	Route for Administration	Rationale
Magnesium gluconate (Magonate)	Orally	Used for mild hypomagnesemia
Magnesium-protein complex (Mg-PLUS)	Orally	Used for mild hypomagnesemia
Magnesium sulfate	Intramuscularly	Used for moderate hypomagnesemia: 1 gram or 2 mL of 50% $MgSO_4$ q8h
	Intravenously	Used for severe hypomagnesemia: 2 grams or 4 mL of 50% $MgSO_4$ diluted in 100 mL of D_5W, administer in 10–15 min

magnesium and calcium. Diuretics, certain antibiotics, laxatives, and steroids are drug groups that promote magnesium loss. An excess intake of magnesium salts is the major cause of serum magnesium excess.

Hypomagnesemia (like hypokalemia) enhances the action of digitalis and causes digitalis toxicity. Magnesium sulfate corrects hypomagnesemia and symptoms of digitalis toxicity. Table 8–8 lists the drugs that affect magnesium balance.

● Clinical Considerations: Magnesium

1. Signs and symptoms of hypomagnesemia are similar to those of hypokalemia.
2. Excess use of laxatives and antacids that contain magnesium can cause hypermagnesemia.
3. A magnesium deficit is often accompanied by a potassium and calcium deficit (40% of clients with hypomagnesemia also have hypokalemia). If a potassium deficit does not respond to potassium replacement, hypomagnesemia should be suspected.
4. Severe hypomagnesemia can cause symptoms of tetany.
5. IV magnesium sulfate diluted in intravenous solution should be administered at a slow rate. Rapid infusion can cause hot and flushed flashes (feeling).

Table 8-8

Drugs Affecting Magnesium Balance

Magnesium Imbalance	Drugs	Rationale

Hypomagnesemia (serum magnesium deficit)	Diuretics
	  Furosemide/Lasix
	  Ethacrynic acid/Edecrin
	  Mannitol
		Diuretics promote urinary loss of magnesium.

	Antibiotics
	  Gentamicin
	  Tobramycin
	  Carbenicillin
	  Capreomycin
	  Neomycin
	  Polymyxin B
	  Amphotericin B
	Digitalis
	Calcium gluconate
	Insulin
		These agents can cause magnesium loss via kidney.

	Laxatives Cisplatin	Laxative abuse causes magnesium loss via GI.

	Corticosteroids
	  Cortisone
	  Prednisone
		Steroids can decrease serum magnesium levels.

Hypermagnesemia (serum magnesium excess)	Magnesium salts:
	Oral and enema
	  Magnesium hydroxide/MOM
	  Magnesium sulfate/Epsom salt
	Magnesium citrate
	Magnesium sulfate (maternity)
		Excess use of magnesium salts can increase serum magnesium levels.
		
		Use of excess $MgSO_4$ in treatment of toxemia can cause hypermagnesemia.

	Lithium	Hypermagnesemia can be associated with lithium therapy.

6. In emergency situations, IV calcium gluconate is given to reverse hypermagnesemia.

7. Long-term administration of saline (NaCl) infusions can result in magnesium and calcium losses. Sodium inhibits renal absorption of magnesium and calcium.

8. A magnesium deficit enhances the action of digoxin.

9. Thiazides and loop (high-ceiling) diuretics decrease serum magnesium levels.

▶ CLIENT MANAGEMENT

Assessment

- Obtain a health history for possible causes of hypomagnesemia or hypermagnesemia; see Tables 8–4 and 8–5.

- Assess for signs and symptoms of hypomagnesemia [tetanylike symptoms (tremors, twitching of the face)] or hypermagnesemia (decreased neuromuscular activity, decreased respiration, and hypotension).

- Obtain a serum magnesium level that can be used as a baseline for comparison of future serum magnesium levels.

- Assess dietary intake and use of intravenous therapy without magnesium. Prolonged intravenous therapy including total parenteral nutrition (TPN) may be a cause of hypomagnesemia.

- Check the ECG/EKG strips for changes. Report abnormal findings.

Diagnoses

- *Altered Nutrition, less than body requirements,* related to poor nutritional intake, chronic alcoholism, chronic laxative abuse, and chronic diarrhea.

- *Altered Nutrition, more than body requirements,* related to oral and intravenous magnesium supplements and chronic use of drugs containing magnesium.

- *Decreased Cardiac Output,* related to a serum magnesium deficit.

Interventions

Hypomagnesemia

- Instruct the client to eat foods rich in magnesium.

- Report when clients receive continuous magnesium-free IV fluids. TPN solutions should contain some magnesium.

- Administer IV magnesium sulfate diluted in IV solution, slowly unless the client has a very severe deficit. Rapid infusion can cause a hot or flushed feeling.

- Have IV calcium gluconate available for emergency to reverse hypermagnesemia from overcorrection.

- Monitor vital signs and ECG strips. Report abnormal findings.
- Report urine output <25 mL/h or 600 mL/day when the client is receiving magnesium supplements. Magnesium excess is excreted by the kidneys.
- Check for positive Trousseau's or Chvostek's signs, indicating severe hypomagnesemia. Tetany symptoms can occur in both magnesium and calcium deficits.

Hypermagnesemia

- Monitor vital signs, ECG strips, and urine output. Report abnormal findings.
- Monitor serum magnesium levels. A serum Mg <1.0 mEq/L or >10 mEq/L can cause a cardiac arrest.
- Instruct client to avoid prolonged use of antacids and laxatives that contain magnesium.
- Suggest that the client increase fluid intake for the purpose of diluting the serum magnesium level unless contraindicated for other health problems.

Evaluation/Outcome

- Evaluate that the cause of the magnesium imbalance has been corrected. Check that serum potassium level is within normal range. Because potassium and magnesium are cations and have similar functions, one electrolyte imbalance affects the other electrolyte balance.
- Evaluate the effect of the therapeutic regimen for the correction of magnesium imbalance; serum magnesium is within normal range.
- Remain free of signs and symptoms of hypomagnesemia or hypermagnesemia; ECG, vital signs, etc., return to the client's normal baseline patterns.

Phosphorus Imbalances

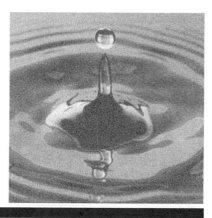

▶ INTRODUCTION

Phosphorus (P) is a major anion that has its highest concentration in the intracellular fluid. Phosphorus and calcium have similar and opposite effects. Both electrolytes need vitamin D for intestinal absorption and are present in bones and teeth. The parathyroid hormone (PTH) acts on phosphorus and calcium differently. PTH decreases serum phosphorus levels by stimulating the renal tubules to excrete phosphorus and increases serum calcium levels by pulling calcium from the bone.

The normal serum phosphorus range is 1.7–2.6 mEq/L or 2.5–4.5 mg/dL. A phosphorus deficit is known as **hypophosphatemia,** and a phosphorus excess is called **hyperphosphatemia.** The ions phosphorus (P) and phosphate (PO_4) are used interchangeably. Phosphorus is measured in the serum, where it appears as the form of phosphate. Forty-five percent of phosphorus is protein-bound and 55% is ionized (free) phosphorus, which is physiologically active. Table 9-1 summarizes the basic information related to phosphorus balance.

Table 9-1

Basic Information Related to Phosphorus Balance

Categories	Phosphorus Data
Distribution	Approximately 85% of phosphorus is located in bones and teeth and 15% is located in the intracellular fluid (ICF).
Functions	For neuromuscular activity, durability of bones and teeth, formation of ATP, utilization of B vitamins, transmission of hereditary traits, metabolism of CHO, proteins, and fats, and as a contributing factor in acid-base balance.
Normal serum values	Phosphorus: 1.7–2.6 mEg/L; 2.5–4.5 mg/dL; 0.81–1.45 mmol/L.
Dietary requirements	Eight hundred to 1200 mg daily.
Food sources	Whole grain, cereal, cheese, milk, eggs, dry beans, beef, pork, fish, poultry, and most carbonated beverages.
Excretion	Ninety percent is excreted via kidneys and 10% is lost via GI secretions.

Phosphorus has many functions. It is a vital element needed in the formation of bones and teeth and for neuromuscular activity. As an essential component of the cell (nucleic acids and cell membrane), it is incorporated into the enzymes needed for metabolism, e.g., adenosine triphosphate (ATP), a transmission of hereditary traits, and acts as an acid-base buffer. Table 9-2 explains the functions of phosphorus.

▶ PATHOPHYSIOLOGY

Hypophosphatemia can occur within 3–4 days after an inadequate nutrient intake. Initially, the kidneys compensate by decreasing urinary phosphate excretion; however, a continuous inadequate intake of phosphorus results in extracellular fluid shift to the cells in order to replace phosphorus loss in the intracellular fluid.

PTH promotes renal excretion of phosphorus (phosphate) and calcium reabsorption. When there is a high serum concentration of phosphorus, aluminum-containing antacids decrease hyperphosphatemia and its symptoms. Hyperphosphatemia causes hypocalcemia.

Table 9-2

Phosphorus and Its Functions

Body Involvement	Functions
Neuromuscular	Normal nerve and muscle activity.
Bones and teeth	Bone and teeth formation, strength, and durability.
Cellular	Formation of high-energy compounds (ATP, ADP). Phosphorus is the backbone of nucleic acids and stores metabolic energy.
	Formation of the red-blood-cell enzyme 2,3-diphosphoglycerate (2,3-DPG) is responsible for delivering oxygen to tissues.
	Utilization of B vitamins.
	Transmission of hereditary traits.
	Metabolism of carbohydrates, proteins, and fats.
	Maintenance of acid-base balance in body fluids.

▶ ETIOLOGY

Dietary changes, gastrointestinal disturbances, hormonal influence, selected drugs, and cellular changes are all associated with hypophosphatemia. Respiratory alkalosis can result from hypophosphatemia. Any carbohydrate-loading diet can cause a phosphorus shift from the serum into the cell, resulting in a decreased serum phosphorus level. Tissue repair following trauma causes phosphorus to shift into the cells.

Excessive use of phosphate supplements and renal insufficiency are factors associated with hyperphosphatemia. Tables 9–3 and 9–4 list the causes of a phosphorus deficit and excess.

▶ CLINICAL MANIFESTATIONS

Clinical manifestations of hypophosphatemia and hyperphosphatemia are determined by the etiology of the phosphorus imbalance. Neuromuscular irregularities, hematologic and cardiopulmonary abnormalities, and abnormal serum phosphorus level are the most common manifestations. Because the symptoms of phosphorus imbalance are often vague, serum values are needed. Table 9-5 (see page 103) lists the clinical manifestations of phosphorus deficit and excess.

Table 9-3

Causes of Hypophosphatemia
(Serum Phosphorus Deficit)

Etiology	Rationale
Dietary Changes	
Malnutrition	Poor nutrition results in a reduction of phosphorus intake.
Chronic alcoholism	Alcoholism contributes to dietary insufficiencies and increased diuresis.
Total parenteral nutrition (TPN, hyperalimentation)	TPN is usually a phosphorus-poor or -free solution. IV concentrated glucose and protein given rapidly shift phosphorus into the cells, thus causing a serum phosphorus deficit.
Gastrointestinal Abnormalities	
Vomiting, anorexia	Loss of phosphorus through the GI tract decreases
Chronic diarrhea	cellular ATP (energy) stores.
Intestinal malabsorption	Vitamin D deficiencies inhibit phosphorus absorption. Phosphorus is absorbed in the jejunum in the presence of vitamin D.
Hormonal Influence	
Hyperparathyroidism (increased PTH)	Parathyroid hormone (PTH) production enhances renal phosphate excretion and calcium reabsorption.
Drug Influence	
Aluminum-containing antacids	Phosphate binds with aluminum to decrease the serum phosphorus level.
Diuretics	Most diuretics promote a decrease in the serum phosphorus level.
Cellular Changes	
Diabetic ketoacidosis	Glycosuria and polyuria increase phosphate excretion. A dextrose infusion with insulin causes a phosphorus shift into the cells; decreasing the serum phosphorus level.
Burns	Phosphorus is lost due to its increased utilization in tissue building.
Acid-base disorders	Respiratory alkalosis from prolonged hyperventilation decreases the serum phosphorus level by causing an intracellular shift of phosphorus. Metabolic alkalosis can also cause this shift.

Table 9-4

Causes of Hyperphosphatemia (Serum Phosphorus Excess)

Etiology	Rationale
Dietary Changes Oral phosphate supplements Intravenous phosphate	Excessive administration of phosphate-containing substances increases the serum phosphorus level.
Hormonal Influence Hypoparathyroidism (lack of PTH)	Lack of PTH causes a calcium loss and a phosphorus excess.
Renal Abnormalities Renal insufficiency	Renal insufficiency or shutdown decreases phosphorus excretion.
Drug Influence Laxatives containing phosphate	Frequent use of phosphate laxatives increases the serum phosphorus level.

▶ CLINICAL MANAGEMENT

When the serum phosphorus level falls below 1.5 mEq/L or 2 mg/dL, oral and/or intravenous phosphate-containing solutions are usually prescribed. If the serum phosphorus level falls below 0.5 mEq/L or 1 mg/dL, severe hypophosphatemia occurs. Intravenous phosphate-containing solutions (sodium phosphate and potassium phosphate) are indicated. Sodium phosphate is the preferred solution if the client has oliguria.

Suggested Phosphorus Replacement for Severe Hypophosphatemia

Uncomplicated P deficit:	IV phosphate salt: 0.6 mg/kg/h
Complicated P deficit:	IV phosphate salt: 0.9 mg/kg/h
Serum P level:	>1.5 mEq/L or 2 mg/dL: oral phosphate salt

Check phosphorus level q6h.

Table 9-5

Clinical Manifestations of Phosphorus Imbalances

Body Involvement	Hypophosphatemia	Hyperphosphatemia
Neuromuscular Abnormalities	Muscle weakness Tremors Paresthesia Bone pain Hyporeflexia Seizures	Tetany (with decreased calcium) Hyperreflexia Flaccid paralysis Muscular weakness
Hematologic Abnormalities	Tissue hypoxia (decreased oxygen-containing hemoglobin and hemolysis) Possible bleeding (platelet dysfunction) Possible infection (leukocyte dysfunction)	
Cardiopulmonary Abnormalities	Weak pulse (myocardial dysfunction) Hyperventilation	Tachycardia
GI Abnormalities	Anorexia Dysphagia	Nausea, diarrhea Abdominal cramps
Laboratory Values Milliequivalents per liter	<1.7 mEq/L	>2.6 mEq/L
Milligrams per deciliter	<2.5 mg/dL	>4.5 mg/dL

Drugs and Their Effect on Phosphorus Balance

The major drug group that causes hypophosphatemia is the aluminum antacids. Other drug groups causing a phosphorus deficit include diuretics, steroids, and calcium salts. Excess use of phosphate laxatives, phosphate enemas, and oral and intravenous phosphates are often responsible for hyperphosphatemia. Table 9-6 lists the drugs that can cause a phosphorus deficit and excess.

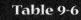

Table 9-6

Drugs That Affect Phosphorus Balance

Phosphorus Imbalance	Drugs	Rationale

Hypophosphatemia (serum phosphorus deficit)	Sucralfate
	Aluminum antacids
	  Amphojel
	  Basaljel
	Aluminum/magnesium
	   antacids
	  Di-Gel
	  Gelusil
	  Maalox
	  Maalox Plus
	  Mylanta
	  Mylanta II
		Aluminum-containing antacids bind with phosphorus; therefore the serum phosphorus level is decreased. Calcium promotes phosphate loss.

	Calcium antacids Calcium carbonate	

	Diuretics
	  Thiazide
	  Loop (high-ceiling)
	  Acetazolamide
		Phosphorus can be lost when diuretics are used.

	Androgens
	Corticosteroids
	  Cortisone
	  Prednisone
	Glucagon
	Gastrin
	Epinephrine
	Mannitol
		These agents have a mild to moderate effect on phosphorus loss.

	Salicylate overdose Insulin and glucose	

continues on the following page

● Clinical Considerations: Phosphorus

1. Phosphorus is needed for durable bones and teeth, formation of ATP (high-energy compound for cellular activity), metabolism of carbohydrates, proteins, and fats, utilization of B vitamins, transmission of hereditary traits, and others.

Table 9-6

(Continued)

Phosphorus Imbalance	Drugs	Rationale

Hyperphosphatemia (serum phosphorus excess)	Oral phosphates
	Sodium phosphate/
	  Phospho-Soda
	Potassium phosphate/
	  Neutra-Phos K
		Excess oral ingestion and IV infusion can increase the serum phosphorus level.

	Intravenous phosphates Sodium phosphate Potassium phosphate	

	Phosphate laxatives
	Sodium phosphate
	Sodium biphosphate/
	  Phospho-Soda
	Phosphate enema
	Fleet sodium
	  phosphate
		Continuous use of phosphate laxatives and enemas can increase the serum phosphorus level.

	Excessive vitamin D
	Antibiotics
	  Tetracyclines
	  Methicillin	

2. Phosphorus and calcium are similar and yet differ in action. Both need vitamin D for intestinal absorption. PTH promotes renal excretion of phosphorus (phosphate) and calcium reabsorption from the bones.

3. Vomiting and chronic diarrhea cause a loss of phosphorus.

4. Concentrated IV phosphates are hyperosmolar (hypertonic) and must be diluted. If IV potassium phosphate is given in intravenous solution, the IV rate should be no more than 10 mEq/h to avoid phlebitis and a potassium overload.

5. Aluminum-containing antacids decrease the serum phosphorus level; phosphate binds with the aluminum. Aluminum-containing antacids are useful for hyperphosphatemia.

6. Continuous use of phosphate laxatives can cause an elevated serum phosphorus level.

▶ CLIENT MANAGEMENT

Assessment

* Obtain a health history of clinical problems associated with hypophosphatemia (malnutrition, chronic alcoholism, chronic diarrhea, vitamin D deficiency, hyperparathyroidism, continuous use of aluminum-containing antacids, and respiratory alkalosis) and with hyperphosphatemia (continuous use of phosphate-containing laxatives, hypoparathyroidism, and renal insufficiency).

* Assess for signs and symptoms of a phosphorus deficit or phosphorus excess (refer to Table 9-5).

* Check the serum phosphorus level. The serum phosphorus level is needed as a baseline level for assessing future serum phosphorus levels.

* Check serum calcium level. An elevated calcium level causes a decreased phosphorus level and vice versa.

* Check vital signs. Report abnormal findings, such as weak pulse, tachypnea.

* Check urinary output. Report abnormal findings. A decrease in urine output, <600 mL/day, increases the serum phosphorus level.

Diagnoses

* *Altered Nutrition, less than body requirements,* related to inadequate nutritional intake, chronic alcoholism, vomiting, chronic diarrhea, lack of vitamin D intake, and intravenous fluids (including TPN), which lack a phosphate additive.

* *Altered Nutrition, more than body requirements,* related to excess intake of phosphate-containing compounds such as some laxatives, intravenous potassium phosphate, and others.

Interventions

Hypophosphatemia

* Monitor serum phosphorus and calcium levels. Report abnormal results.

* Monitor oral and intravenous phosphate replacements. An oral phosphate salt, Neutrophos, which comes in capsules, may be indicated if nausea is present. Administer IV potassium phosphate slowly to prevent hyperphosphatemia and irritation of the blood vessel. Rapid intravenous potassium phosphate can cause phlebitis.

- Check for signs of infiltration at the IV site; KPO_4 is extremely irritating to the subcutaneous tissue and can cause sloughing of tissue and necrosis.

- Encourage the client to eat foods rich in phosphorus, such as meats, milk, whole grain cereal, and nuts. Most carbonated drinks are high in phosphates.

- Instruct the client to avoid taking antacids that contain aluminum hydroxide, such as Amphojel. Phosphorus binds with aluminum products; a low serum phosphorus level results.

Hyperphosphatemia

- Monitor vital signs. Report abnormal results.

- Monitor serum phosphorus and calcium levels. Report abnormal results.

- Observe the client for signs and symptoms of hypocalcemia (e.g., tetany). An increased serum phosphorus level decreases the calcium level.

- Monitor urine output. Report inadequate urine output. Phosphorus is excreted by the kidneys and poor renal function can cause hyperphosphatemia.

- Instruct the client to eat foods that are low in phosphorus and to avoid carbonated beverages, which are high in phosphorus.

Evaluation/Outcome

- Evaluate that the cause of phosphorus imbalance has been eliminated.

- Evaluate the effect of clinical management in the correction of hypophosphatemia or hyperphosphatemia; serum phosphorus levels are within normal range.

- Determine that the signs and symptoms of phosphorus imbalance are absent; client is free of neuromuscular abnormalities, such as muscle weakness and tetany symptoms.

- Document compliance with prescribed drug therapy and medical and dietary regimen.

Acid-Base Balance and Imbalance

▶ INTRODUCTION

Our body fluid must maintain a balance between acidity and alkalinity in order for life to be maintained. The concentration of hydrogen ions (plus or minus) determine either the acidity or the alkalinity of a solution. The amount of ionized hydrogen in extracellular fluid is extremely small: around 0.0000001 g/L. The pH symbol stands for the negative logarithm of the hydrogen ion concentration. Mathematically, it is expressed as 10^{-7}. When the minus sign is dropped, the symbol is used to designate the hydrogen ion concentration as pH 7. As the hydrogen ion concentration rises in solution, the pH value falls, thus indicating increased acidity. As the hydrogen ion concentration falls, the pH rises, thus indicating increased alkalinity.

The hydroxyl ions (OH^-) are base ions and, when in excess, increase the alkalinity of the solution. A solution with a pH 7 is neutral since at this concentration the number of hydrogen ions is exactly balanced with the number of hydroxyl ions.

The pH of extracellular fluid in a healthy individual is maintained at a level between 7.35 and 7.45, resulting in a body fluid level that is slightly alkaline. If the pH value is below 7.35, acidosis is present, and if the pH value exceeds 7.45, alkalosis results. Within the body, the pH of the different body fluids varies. Table U3-1 lists the various body fluids and their pH ranges.

In health, there are $1\frac{1}{3}$ mEq/L of acid to each 27 mEq of alkali for each liter of extracellular fluid. This represents a ratio of 1 part acid to 20 parts alkali. Figure U3-1 demonstrates by the arrow that the body is in acid-base balance; a pH of 7.4 represents this balance. If the arrow tilts left due to an alkali deficit or acid excess, then acidosis occurs. If the arrow tilts right due to an alkali excess or acid deficit, then alkalosis occurs.

Table U3-1

The pH of Body Fluids

Body Fluid	pH
Extracellular fluid	7.35–7.45
Intracellular fluid	6.9–7.2
Urine	6.0
Gastric juice	1.0–2.0
Intestinal juice	6.6–7.6
Bile	5.0–6.0

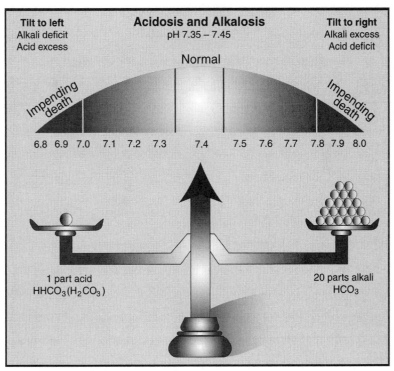

Figure U3-1 Acidosis and Alkalosis

▶ REGULATORY MECHANISMS FOR pH CONTROL

The four major regulatory mechanisms for pH control are:

1. Buffer systems
2. Ion exchange
3. Respiratory regulation
4. Renal regulation

The buffer systems maintain the acid-base balance of body fluids by protecting the fluids against changes in pH. The most important buffer system in the body is the bicarbonate–carbonic acid buffer which maintains the acid-base balance 55% of the time. Table U3-2 provides specific data related to the regulation of pH control in regards to the four major regulatory mechanisms.

Table U3-2

Regulatory Mechanism for pH Control

Regulatory Mechanism	Intervention
Buffer Systems a. Bicarbonate–carbonic acid buffer system (principal buffer system of body)	Acids combine with bicarbonates in blood to form neutral salts (bicarbonate salt) and carbonic acid (weak acid). Carbonic acid (H_2CO_3) is weak and unstable acid, changing to water and carbon dioxide in fluid ($H_2CO_3 \rightleftharpoons H_2O + CO_2$). A strong base combines with weak acid, e.g., H_2CO_3.
b. Phosphate buffer system	The phosphate buffer system increases the amount of sodium bicarbonate ($NaHCO_3$) in extracellular fluids, making extracellular fluids more alkaline. The H^+ is excreted as NaH_2PO_4 and Na and bicarbonate ions combine.

continues on the following page

Table U3-2

(Continued)

Regulatory Mechanism	Intervention
c. Hemoglobin-oxyhemoglobin buffer system	Maintains same pH level in venous blood as in arterial blood.
d. Protein buffer system	Proteins can exist in form of acids (H protein) or alkaline salts (B protein) and in this way are able to bind or release excess hydrogen as required.
Ion exchange	Ion exchange of HCO_3 and Cl occurs in red blood cells (RBCs) as result of O_2 and CO_2 exchange. There is redistribution of anions in response to increase in CO_2. Chloride ion enters RBCs as bicarbonate ion and diffuses into plasma in order to restore ionic balance.
Respiratory regulation (acts quickly in case of emergency)	For regulation of acid balance, the lungs blow off more CO_2, and for regulation of alkaline balance, the respiratory center depresses respirations in order to retain CO_2. It takes 1–3 minutes for the respiratory system to readjust H^+ concentration.
Renal Regulation a. Acidification of phosphate buffer salts	Exchange mechanism occurs between H^+ of renal tubular cells and disodium salt (Na_2HPO_4) in tubular urine.
b. Reabsorption of bicarbonate	Carbon dioxide is absorbed by tubular cells from blood and combines with water present in cells to form carbonic acid, which in turn ionizes, forming H^+ and HCO_3^-. Na^+ of tubular urine exchanges with H^+ of tubular cells and combines with HCO_3^- to form sodium bicarbonate and is reabsorbed into blood.
c. Secretion of ammonia	Ammonia (NH_3) unites with HCl in renal tubules and H^+ is excreted as NH_4Cl (ammonium chloride).

Determination of Acid-Base Imbalances

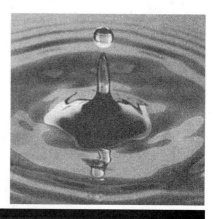

▶ INTRODUCTION

Hydrogen ions circulate throughout the body fluids in two forms, *volatile acid* and *nonvolatile acid.* A volatile acid (carbonic acid [H_2CO_3]) circulates as CO_2 and H_2O and is excreted as a gas, CO_2. A nonvolatile acid (fixed acid, e.g., lactic, pyruvic, sulfuric, phosphoric acids) is from the various organic acids within the body. It is excreted from the body in urine. The lungs and the kidneys aid in the regulation of acid-base balance; the lungs excrete the volatile acid and the kidneys excrete nonvolatile acids. The formula that demonstrates respiratory and renal regulation for acid-base balance is shown in Figure 10-1.

Arterial blood gases are drawn to determine acid-base imbalance. The three values (pH, $PaCO_2$, and HCO_3) are analyzed from the arterial blood specimen to indicate the type of acid-base imbalance. The pH indicates either that the extracellular fluid is neutral (7.35–7.45), acidotic (<7.35) or alkalotic (>7.45). $PaCO_2$ is the respiratory component for checking acid-base imbalance. If the $PaCO_2$ is >45 mm Hg,

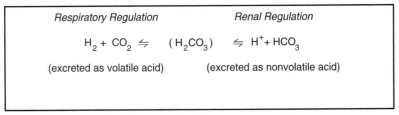

Respiratory Regulation	Renal Regulation
$H_2 + CO_2 \leftrightarrows (H_2CO_3) \leftrightarrows H^+ + HCO_3$	
(excreted as volatile acid)	(excreted as nonvolatile acid)

Figure 10-1 Respiratory and Renal Regulation of Acid-Base Balance

respiratory acidosis occurs; if $PaCO_2$ is <35 mm Hg, respiratory alkalosis is present. The metabolic or renal component is HCO_3. If the HCO_3 is <24 mEq/L, metabolic acidosis occurs; if it is >28 mEq/L, metabolic alkalosis is present. Other measurements to determine metabolic acidosis and alkalosis are base excess (BE) and serum CO_2, a serum bicarbonate determinant. The norm for base excess is −2 to +2. BE relates to the bicarbonate range of 24 to 28 mEq/L, with a BE norm of 26 mEq/L (−2 = 24 mEq/L and +2 = 28 mEq/L). Table 10-1 presents the normal values for these tests and the types of acid-base imbalances that occur.

To determine the type of acid-base imbalance:

1. pH should be checked first. If it is less than 7.35, acidosis is present. If it is greater than 7.45, alkalosis is present.

2. $PaCO_2$ is checked next. If it is within normal range, respiratory acidosis or alkalosis is *not* occurring. If the $PaCO_2$ is greater than 45 mm Hg and the pH is less than 7.35, respiratory acidosis occurs.

3. HCO_3 is checked. If the bicarbonate is less than 24 mEq/L and the pH is less than 7.35, metabolic acidosis is present.

Figure 10–2 outlines the method for determining acid-base imbalances.

▶ COMPENSATION FOR pH BALANCE

There are specific compensatory reactions in response to metabolic acidosis and alkalosis and to respiratory acidosis and alkalosis. The pH returns to normal or close to normal by changing the component ($PaCO_2$ or HCO_3) that originally was *not* affected.

The respiratory system can compensate for metabolic acidosis and alkalosis. In metabolic acidosis, the lungs (stimulated by the respiratory center) hyperventilate to decrease the CO_2 level; the $PaCO_2$ decreases due to "blowing off" of carbon dioxide and water, which decreases the body's carbonic acid (H_2CO_3) level. An example of respiratory compensation is pH 7.33, $PaCO_2$ 32 mm Hg, and HCO_3 18 mEq/L. The pH shows slight acidosis, and the HCO_3 is definitely low, confirming metabolic acidosis.

Table 10-1

Determination of Acid-Base Imbalance

Blood Tests	Normal Values	Imbalance
pH	Adult: 7.35–7.45 Newborn: 7.27–7.47 Child: 7.33–7.43	Adult: <7.35 = acidosis >7.45 = alkalosis

$PaCO_2$
(respiratory
  component)
	Adult and child:
	  35–45 mm Hg
	Newborn:
	  27–41 mm Hg
		Adult and child:
		  <35 mm Hg = respiratory
		  alkalosis (hyperventilation)
		  >45 mm Hg = respiratory
		  acidosis (hypoventilation)

HCO_3^-
(metabolic and renal
  component)
	Adult and child:
	  24–28 mEq/L
	Newborn:
	  22–30 mEq/L
		Adult and child:
		  <24 mEq/L = metabolic acidosis
		  >28 mEq/L = metabolic alkalosis

Base excess (BE)
(metabolic and renal
  component)
	Adult and child
	  +2 to −2
		Adult and child
		  <-2 = metabolic acidosis
		  $>+2$ = metabolic alkalosis

CO_2*
(metabolic and renal
  component)
	Adult and child:
	  22–32 mEq/L
		Adult and child:
		  <22 mEq/L = metabolic acidosis
		  >32 mEq/L = metabolic alkalosis

*Serum CO_2 is a serum bicarbonate determinant and is frequently called *CO_2 combining power.* It refers to the amount of cations, e.g., H^+, Na^+, K^+, etc., available to combine with HCO_3^-. The level of HCO_3^- in the blood is determined by the amount of CO_2 dissolved in the blood.

The $PaCO_2$ should be normal (35 to 45 mm Hg); however, it is low because the respiratory center compensates for the acidotic state by "blowing off" CO_2 (hyperventilating); respiratory compensation occurs. Without this compensation, the pH would be extremely low; e.g., pH of 7.2.

The renal system can compensate for respiratory acidosis and alkalosis. With respiratory acidosis, the kidneys excrete more acid, H^+, and conserve HCO_3. With a pH of 7.34, $PaCO_2$ of 68, and HCO_3 of 35, the pH reveals a slight acidosis and the $PaCO_2$ is highly elevated, indicating CO_2 retention (carbon dioxide and water = carbonic acid) and respiratory acidosis. The HCO_3 indicates renal or metabolic compensation. Without this compensation, the pH would be lower.

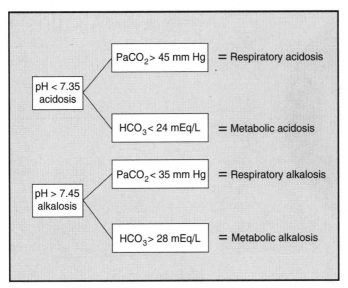

Figure 10-2 Types of Acid-Base Imbalances

● Clinical Considerations: Determination of Acid-Base Imbalances

1. Hydrogen ions circulate in the body fluid in the form of a volatile acid (carbonic acid [H_2CO_3]). The volatile acid is excreted as a gas, CO_2, from the lungs, and the nonvolatile acid (fixed acid; e.g., lactic, pyruvic, ketones), which is excreted in the urine. The lungs and kidneys regulate the hydrogen ions; thus, lung and kidney disorders can cause an acid-base imbalance.

2. To determine acid-base imbalance, the pH should be checked first. The pH determines if the body fluids are within normal range (7.35–7.45), acidotic (<7.35) or alkalotic (>7.45).

3. To determine metabolic acidosis or metabolic alkalosis, first check the pH, then the bicarbonate (HCO_3). If the pH is <7.35 and the HCO_3 is <24 mEq/L, the acid-base imbalance is metabolic acidosis. If the pH is >7.45 and the HCO_3 is >28 mEq/L, metabolic alkalosis is occurring.

4. To determine the presence of respiratory acidosis or respiratory alkalosis, first check the pH, and then the $PaCO_2$. If the pH is <7.35 and the $PaCO_2$ is >45 mm Hg, the acid-base imbalance is respiratory acidosis. If the pH is >7.45 and $PaCO_2$ <35 mm Hg, respiratory alkalosis is occurring.

Metabolic Acidosis and Metabolic Alkalosis

CHAPTER

11

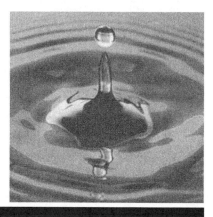

▌ INTRODUCTION

The metabolic/renal components for metabolic acidosis and alkalosis include arterial bicarbonate (HCO_3), base excess (BE), and serum CO_2. In metabolic acidosis, the pH is decreased, or <7.35, the HCO_3 is <24 mEq/L, and the base excess (BE) is <−2. In metabolic alkalosis, the pH is increased or >7.45, the HCO_3 is >28 mEq/L, and the BE is >+2.

▌ PATHOPHYSIOLOGY

Metabolic acidosis is characterized by a decrease in bicarbonate concentration or acid excess. With metabolic alkalosis, there is an increase in bicarbonate concentration or a loss of the hydrogen ion (strong acid) in the extracellular fluid.

Anion gap is a useful indicator for determining the presence or absence of metabolic acidosis. The anion gap can be obtained by using the following formula.

Serum sodium (Na)	–	Serum chloride	+	Serum CO_2	=	Anion gap
Example: 142 mEq/L	–	102 mEq/L	+	18 mEq/L	=	
142	–	120			=	22 mEq/L

If the anion gap is >16 mEq/L, metabolic acidosis is suspected. According to the example, the anion gap is 22 mEq/L, so metabolic acidosis is present.

Conditions associated with an anion gap that is greater than 16 mEq/L are diabetic ketoacidosis, lactic acidosis, poisoning, and renal failure. If a client takes excessive amounts of baking soda or commercially prepared acid neutralizers to ease indigestion or stomach ulcer pain, the anion gap is much less than 16 mEq/L, so the imbalance results in metabolic alkalosis.

▶ ETIOLOGY

The causes of metabolic acidosis include starvation, severe malnutrition, chronic diarrhea, kidney failure, diabetic ketoacidosis, hyperthyroidism, thyrotoxicosis, trauma, shock, excessive exercise, severe infection, and prolonged fever. Table 11-1 describes the causes and rationale for each disorder. In metabolic alkalosis, typical etiologic factors include vomiting, gastric suction, peptic ulcers, and hypokalemia. Table 11-2 describes each cause and rationale.

▶ CLINICAL MANIFESTATIONS

When metabolic acidosis occurs, the central nervous system (CNS) is depressed. Symptoms can include apathy, disorientation, weakness, and stupor. Deep rapid breathing is a respiratory compensatory mechanism for decreasing the acid content in the blood.

In metabolic alkalosis, excitability of the CNS occurs. These symptoms may include irritability, mental confusion, tetanylike symptoms, and hyperactive reflexes. Hypoventilation may occur as a compensatory mechanism for metabolic alkalosis to conserve the hydrogen ions and carbonic acid. Table 11-3 lists the clinical manifestations related to metabolic acidosis and alkalosis.

In metabolic acidosis, the renal and respiratory mechanisms try to reestablish the pH balance. The H^+ exchanges with the Na^+, and thus H^+ is excreted in the urine. Kussmaul breathing (rapid deep breathing) causes CO_2 to be blown off through the lungs, decreasing carbonic acid (H_2CO_3) levels.

Table 11-1

Causes of Metabolic Acidosis

Etiology	Rationale
Gastrointestinal Abnormalities	
Starvation	Nonvolatile acids, i.e., lactic and pyruvic acids, occur
Severe malnutrition	as the result of an accumulation of acid products from cellular breakdown due to starvation and/or severe malnutrition.
Chronic diarrhea	Loss of bicarbonate ions in the small intestines is in excess. Also, the loss of sodium ions exceeds that of chloride ions. Cl^- combines with H^+, producing a strong acid (HCl).
Renal Abnormalities	
Kidney failure	Kidney mechanisms for conserving sodium and water and for excreting H^+ fail.
Hormonal Influence	
Diabetic ketoacidosis	Failure to metabolize adequate quantities of glucose causes the liver to increase metabolism of fatty acids. Oxidation of fatty acids produces ketone bodies, which cause the ECF to become more acid. Ketones require a base for excretion.
Hyperthyroidism, thyrotoxicosis	An overactive thyroid gland can cause cellular catabolism (breakdown) due to a severe increase in metabolism, which increases cellular needs.
Others	
Trauma, shock	Trauma and shock cause cellular breakdown and the release of nonvolatile acids.
Excess exercise, severe infection, fever	Excessive exercise, fever, and severe infection can cause cellular catabolism and acid accumulation.

In metabolic alkalosis, the buffer, renal, and respiratory mechanisms try to reestablish balance. With the buffer mechanism, the excess bicarbonate reacts with buffer acid salts to decrease the number of bicarbonate ions in the extracellular fluid and increase the concentration of carbonic acid. The renal mechanism functions by conserving the hydrogen ions and excreting the sodium, potassium, and bicarbonate ions. The respiratory mechanism maintains balance through hypoventilation, retaining carbon dioxide and increasing the concentration of carbonic acid in the extracellular fluid.

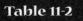

Table 11-2

Causes of Metabolic Alkalosis

Etiology	Rationale
Gastrointestinal Abnormalities	
Vomiting, gastric suction	With vomiting and gastric suctioning, large amounts of chloride and hydrogen ions that are plentiful in the stomach are lost. Bicarbonate anions increase to compensate for chloride loss.
Peptic ulcers	Excess of alkali in ECF occurs when a client takes excessive amounts of acid neutralizers such as $NaHCO_3$ to ease ulcer pain.
Hypokalemia	Loss of potassium from the body is accompanied by loss of chloride.

Table 11-3

Clinical Manifestations of Metabolic Acidosis and Metabolic Alkalosis

Body Involvement	Metabolic Acidosis	Metabolic Alkalosis
CNS Abnormalities	Restlessness, apathy, weakness, disorientation, stupor, coma	Irritability, confusion, tetanylike symptoms, hyperactive reflexes
Respiratory Abnormalities	Kussmaul breathing: deep, rapid, vigorous breathing	Shallow breathing
Skin Changes	Flushing and warm skin	
Cardiac Abnormalities	Cardiac dysrhythmias, decrease in heart rate and cardiac output	
Gastrointestinal Abnormalities	Nausea, vomiting, abdominal pain	Vomiting with loss of chloride and potassium
Laboratory Values		
pH	<7.35	>7.45
HCO_3, BE	<24 mEq/L; <−2	>28 mEq/L; >+2
Serum CO_2	<22 mEq/L	>32 mEq/L

▶ CLINICAL MANAGEMENT

The first line of treatment for metabolic acidosis and alkalosis is to determine the cause of the imbalance. Correcting the cause may completely alleviate the symptoms. Giving fluids intravenously and restoring electrolytes and nutrients assist by correcting metabolic acid-base imbalances. Figure 11-1 outlines the body's normal defense actions and various methods of treatment for restoring balance in metabolic acidosis and alkalosis.

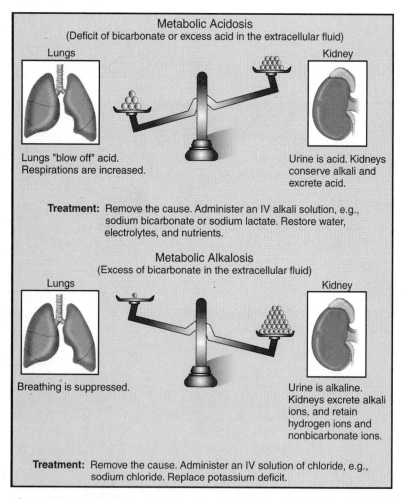

Figure 11-1 Body's Defense Action and Treatment for Metabolic Acidosis and Alkalosis

● Clinical Considerations: Metabolic Acidosis and Alkalosis

1. Metabolic acidosis is characterized by a decrease in bicarbonate concentration or acid excess. The pH is <7.35, HCO_3 is <24 mEq/L, base excess (BE) is <−2.

2. The anion gap is a useful indicator for determining the presence or absence of metabolic acidosis. If the anion gap is >16 mEq/L, metabolic acidosis is suspected. The formula used is: Serum sodium − Serum chloride + Serum CO_2 = Anion gap

3. With metabolic acidosis, the CNS is depressed; symptoms include apathy, disorientation, weakness, and stupor. Deep rapid breathing (Kussmaul breathing) is a respiratory compensatory mechanism to decrease acid content in the blood.

4. Metabolic alkalosis is characterized by an increase in bicarbonate concentration or a loss of a strong acid (hydrogen ion). The pH is >7.45, HCO_3 is >28 mEq/L, BE >+2.

5. Vomiting, gastric suction, and ingestion of large amounts of a sodium bicarbonate preparation are common causes of metabolic alkalosis.

6. In metabolic alkalosis, the buffer, renal, and respiratory mechanisms try to reestablish balance. The renal mechanism functions by conserving hydrogen ions, and excreting sodium, potassium, and bicarbonate. Hypoventilation is a respiratory compensatory mechanism, which retains CO_2, thus increasing the carbonic acid (H_2CO_3) concentration.

▶ CLIENT MANAGEMENT

Assessment

- Obtain a client history of current clinical problems. Identify health problems associated with metabolic acidosis, such as starvation, severe or chronic diarrhea, diabetic ketoacidosis, trauma and shock, kidney failure, and problems associated with metabolic alkalosis, such as vomiting, gastric suction, peptic ulcer.

- Check the arterial bicarbonate, base excess, and serum CO_2 levels for metabolic acid-base imbalances. Compare with the norms for arterial blood gases.

- Obtain baseline vital signs for comparison with future vital signs.

- Check laboratory results, especially blood sugar and electrolytes.

Diagnoses

- *Altered Nutrition less than body requirements,* related to starvation, diabetic ketoacidosis, and so on.
- *Decreased Cardiac Output,* related to severe metabolic acidotic state.
- *Fluid Volume Deficit,* related to vomiting or nasogastric suctioning.

Interventions

Metabolic Acidosis

- Monitor dietary intake and report inadequate nutrient and fluid intake.
- Report abnormal laboratory results regarding electrolytes, blood sugar, and arterial blood gases (ABGs). A pH <7.35 and HCO_3 <24 mEq/L indicate metabolic acidosis.
- Monitor vital signs. Report the presence of Kussmaul respirations that relate to diabetic ketoacidosis or severe shock.
- Monitor signs and symptoms related to metabolic acidosis (refer to Table 11-3).
- Monitor fluid intake and output. Report the amount of fluid loss via vomiting and gastric suctioning.
- Administer adequate fluid replacement with sodium bicarbonate as prescribed by the health care provider to correct acidotic state.

Metabolic Alkalosis

- Monitor serum electrolytes and ABG values. A pH >7.45 and HCO_3 >28 mEq/L indicate metabolic alkalosis.
- Monitor vital signs. Note if the respirations remain shallow and slow.
- Monitor signs and symptoms of metabolic alkalosis (refer to Table 11-3).
- Report the consumption of large quantities of acid neutralizers that contain bicarbonate compounds such as Bromo-Seltzer.
- Record the amount of fluid loss via vomiting and gastric suctioning. Hydrogen and chloride are lost with the gastric secretions, thus the pH is increased and metabolic alkalosis results.
- Provide comfort and alleviate anxiety when possible.

Evaluation/Outcome

- Evaluate that the cause of metabolic acidosis or metabolic alkalosis has been corrected or controlled.

- Evaluate the therapeutic effect on the correction of metabolic acidosis or metabolic alkalosis; ABGs are returning to or have returned to normal range.

- Remain free of signs and symptoms of metabolic acidosis or metabolic alkalosis; vital signs returned to normal range, especially respiration.

- Client is able to perform activities of daily living.

Respiratory Acidosis and Respiratory Alkalosis

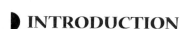

▶ INTRODUCTION

The $PaCO_2$ is the respiratory component that determines respiratory acidosis and alkalosis. In respiratory acidosis, the CO_2 is conserved by mixing it with water to form carbonic acid (H_2CO_3). In respiratory acidosis, the pH is decreased (<7.35) and the $PaCO_2$ is increased (>45 mm Hg). In respiratory alkalosis, the pH is increased (>7.45) and the $PaCO_2$ is decreased (<35 mm Hg).

▶ PATHOPHYSIOLOGY

Respiratory acidosis is characterized by an increase in carbon dioxide and carbonic acid concentration in the extracellular fluid. Respiratory alkalosis is characterized by a decrease in carbon dioxide and carbonic acid in the extracellular fluid. Figure 12-1 demonstrates the relationship of the pH to the $PaCO_2$. When the pH is decreased and the $PaCO_2$ is increased, respiratory acidosis occurs. Likewise, if the pH is increased and the $PaCO_2$ is decreased, respiratory alkalosis occurs.

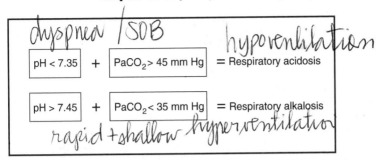

dyspnea /SOB   *hypoventilation*

| pH < 7.35 | + | PaCO$_2$> 45 mm Hg | = Respiratory acidosis |

| pH > 7.45 | + | PaCO$_2$< 35 mm Hg | = Respiratory alkalosis |

rapid +shallow hyperventilation

Figure 12-1 Relationship of pH and PaCO$_2$ in Respiratory Acid-Base Imbalances

Very often, inadequate ventilation is the cause of respiratory acidosis. The characteristic breathing pattern associated with respiratory acidosis is dyspnea or shortness of breath because hypoventilation usually causes a decrease in the PaCO$_2$. In respiratory alkalosis, breathing is rapid and shallow (hyperventilation). In respiratory acidosis, the buffer, renal, and respiratory mechanisms try to reestablish balance. As a result of a chloride shift, bicarbonate ions are released to neutralize carbonic acid excess. In respiratory alkalosis, the buffer mechanism produces more organic acids which react with the excess bicarbonate ions. There is an increase in bicarbonate excretion and a retention of the hydrogen ion.

▶ ETIOLOGY

Inadequate exchange of gases in the lungs causes a retention of CO$_2$ and carbonic acid in the blood (CO$_2$ + H$_2$O = H$_2$CO$_3$), resulting in respiratory acidosis. Respiratory alkalosis results from a CO$_2$ loss, lungs blowing off carbon dioxide. Tables 12-1 and 12-2 list the causes of respiratory acidosis and alkalosis.

Narcotics, sedatives, chest injuries, respiratory distress syndrome, pneumonia, and pulmonary edema can cause acute respiratory acidosis (ARA). ARA results from rapidly increasing CO$_2$ levels and retention of CO$_2$ in the blood. With chronic obstructive pulmonary disease (COPD), the PaCO$_2$ gradually increases over a prolonged period of time (days to months). The body can compensate for CO$_2$ accumulation by excreting excess hydrogen ions and conserving the bicarbonate ion. The client's PaCO$_2$ can be extremely elevated and the HCO$_3$ also elevated, indicating metabolic/renal compensation. An example of compensated ABG for a client with COPD is pH 7.22, PaCO$_2$ 98 mm Hg, HCO$_3$ 40. Refer to Chapter 10 for a discussion of acid-base compensation mechanisms.

Those in respiratory alkalosis are often very apprehensive and anxious. They hyperventilate to overcome their anxiety. This causes them to blow off excessive quantities of carbon dioxide, which results in a respiratory alkalotic state.

Table 12-1

Causes of Respiratory Acidosis

Etiology	Rationale
CNS Depressants Drugs: narcotics [morphine, meperidine (Demerol)], anesthetics, barbiturates	These drugs depress the respiratory center in the medulla, causing retention of CO_2 (carbon dioxide), which results in hypercapnia (increased partial pressure of CO_2 in the blood).
Pulmonary Abnormalities Chronic obstructive pulmonary disease (COPD: emphysema, severe asthma)	Inadequate exchange of gases in the lungs due to a decreased surface area for aeration causes retention of CO_2 in the blood.
Pneumonia, pulmonary edema	Airway obstruction inhibits effective gas exchanges, resulting in a retention of CO_2.
Poliomyelitis, Guillain-Barré syndrome, chest injuries	Weakness of the respiratory muscles decreases the excretion of CO_2, thus increasing carbonic acid concentration.

Table 12-2

Causes of Respiratory Alkalosis

Etiology	Rationale
Hyperventilation Psychologic effects: anxiety, hysteria, overbreathing Pain	Excessive "blowing off" CO_2 through the lungs results in hypocapnia (decreased partial pressure of CO_2 in the blood).
Fever Brain tumors, meningitis, encephalitis	Overstimulation of the respiratory center in the medulla results in hyperventilation.
Early salicylate poisoning Hyperthyroidism	

▶ CLINICAL MANIFESTATIONS

In respiratory acidosis, an increase in hypercapnia causes dyspnea (difficulty in breathing), an increased pulse rate, and an elevated blood pressure. The skin may be warm and flushed due to vasodilation from the increased CO_2 concentration.

Table 12-3

Clinical Manifestations of Respiratory Acidosis and Respiratory Alkalosis

Body Involvement	Respiratory Acidosis	Respiratory Alkalosis
Cardiopulmonary Abnormalities	Dyspnea Tachycardia Blood pressure	Rapid, shallow breathing Palpitations
CNS Abnormalities	Disorientation Depression, paranoia Weakness Stupor (later)	Tetany symptoms: numbness and tingling of fingers and toes, positive Chvostek's and Trousseau's signs Hyperactive reflexes Vertigo (dizziness) Unconsciousness (later)
Skin	Flushed and warm	Sweating may occur
Laboratory Values pH	<7.35 (when compensatory mechanisms fail)	>7.45 (when compensatory mechanisms fail)
$PaCO_2$	>45 mm Hg	<35 mm Hg

When respiratory alkalosis occurs, there is CNS hyperexcitability and a decrease in cerebral blood flow. Tetanylike symptoms and dizziness frequently result. Table 12-3 lists the signs and symptoms of respiratory acidosis and alkalosis.

▶ CLINICAL MANAGEMENT

The three treatment modalities for respiratory acidosis are: remove the cause; have the client perform deep breathing exercises; use a ventilator. In respiratory acidosis, the kidneys conserve alkali and excrete hydrogen or acid in the urine. Excess CO_2 accumulation stimulates the lungs to blow off carbon dioxide or acid to compensate for the respiratory acidotic state.

With respiratory alkalosis, the three treatment modalities include: remove the cause; have the client rebreathe expired air to obtain CO_2; use antianxiety drugs. The kidneys excrete alkaline ions (HCO_3) and retain acid or hydrogen ions. Figure 12-2 demonstrates the body's defense action and treatment for respiratory acidosis and alkalosis.

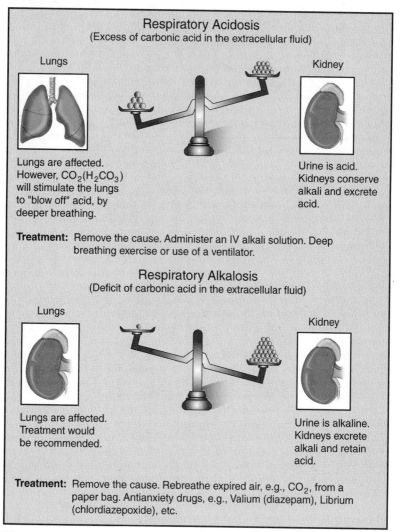

Respiratory Acidosis
(Excess of carbonic acid in the extracellular fluid)

Lungs

Kidney

Lungs are affected.
However, $CO_2(H_2CO_3)$
will stimulate the lungs
to "blow off" acid, by
deeper breathing.

Urine is acid.
Kidneys conserve
alkali and excrete
acid.

Treatment: Remove the cause. Administer an IV alkali solution. Deep
breathing exercise or use of a ventilator.

Respiratory Alkalosis
(Deficit of carbonic acid in the extracellular fluid)

Lungs

Kidney

Lungs are affected.
Treatment would
be recommended.

Urine is alkaline.
Kidneys excrete
alkali and retain
acid.

Treatment: Remove the cause. Rebreathe expired air, e.g., CO_2, from a
paper bag. Antianxiety drugs, e.g., Valium (diazepam), Librium
(chlordiazepoxide), etc.

Figure 12-2 Body's Defense Action and Treatment for Respiratory Acidosis and
Alkalosis

● Clinical Considerations: Respiratory Acidosis and Alkalosis

1. Respiratory acidosis is characterized by an increase in CO_2 and
   H_2CO_3 concentration in body fluids. The pH is <7.35 and $PaCO_2$
   >45 mm Hg.

2. ABG should be closely monitored when respiratory acidosis is suspected; e.g., with chest injuries, respiratory distress syndrome, COPD (asthma, emphysema, chronic bronchitis), pneumonia.

3. Warm, flushed skin (vasodilation from increased CO_2), dyspnea, increased pulse rate are signs and symptoms of respiratory acidosis due to hypercapnia.

4. Respiratory alkalosis is characterized by a decrease in CO_2 and H_2CO_3 concentration in body fluids. The pH is >7.45 and $PaCO_2 < 35$ mm Hg.

5. Severe apprehension and anxiety leads to hyperventilation and respiratory alkalosis. Dizziness and tetanylike symptoms occur.

6. Treatment modalities include rebreathing expired air via paper bag (not plastic bag) and use of antianxiety drugs.

▶ CLIENT MANAGEMENT

Assessment

- Obtain a client history of clinical problems. Identify health problems associated with respiratory acidosis and alkalosis (refer to Tables 12-1 and 12-2).

- Check for signs and symptoms of respiratory acidosis and alkalosis (refer to Table 12-3).

- Obtain vital signs for a baseline record to compare with future vital signs.

- Check arterial blood gases (ABG), particularly the pH and $PaCO_2$. A pH <7.35 and $PaCO_2 > 45$ mm Hg are indicative of respiratory acidosis; a pH >7.45 and $PaCO_2 < 35$ mm Hg are indicative of respiratory alkalosis.

Diagnoses

- *Impaired Gas Exchange,* related to inadequate ventilation (hypoventilation) secondary to COPD.

- *Ineffective Airway Clearance,* related to thick bronchial secretions and/or bronchial spasms.

- *Risk for Injury,* related to hypoxemia and hypercapnia.

- *Ineffective Breathing Pattern,* related to inadequate ventilation.

- *Ineffective Breathing Pattern,* related to hyperventilation and anxiety.

- *Risk for Injury,* related to dizziness, lightheadedness, and syncope secondary to respiratory alkalosis (hyperventilating).

Interventions

Respiratory Acidosis

- Monitor the client's respiratory status for changes in respiratory rate, distress, and breathing pattern.
- Monitor arterial blood gases.
- Auscultate breath sounds periodically to determine wheezing, rhonchi, or crackles (rales) that indicate poor gas exchange.
- Monitor vital signs for tachycardia or cardiac dysrhythmias associated with hypercapnia and hypoxemia (oxygen deficit in the blood).
- Encourage the client to breathe deeply and cough to eliminate bronchial secretions and improve gas exchange.
- Assist the client with use of an inhaler containing a bronchodilator drug.
- Administer chest clapping on COPD clients to break up mucous plugs and secretions in the alveoli.
- Teach breathing exercises and postural drainage to clients with COPD to remove secretions that are trapped in overextended alveoli.
- Encourage the client to increase fluid intake in order to decrease tenacity of secretions.
- Monitor the client's state of sensorium for signs of disorientation due to a lack of oxygen to the brain.
- Encourage the client to participate in a pulmonary rehabilitation program.

Respiratory Alkalosis

- Encourage the client who is overanxious and hyperventilating to take deep breaths and breathe slowly to prevent respiratory alkalosis.
- Listen to the client who is emotionally distressed. Encourage the client to seek professional help.
- Demonstrate a slow, relaxed breathing pattern to decrease over-breathing, which causes respiratory alkalosis.

- Administer a sedative as prescribed to relax the client and restore a normal breathing pattern.
- Monitor ABG and vital signs.

Evaluation/Outcome

- Evaluate that the cause of respiratory acidosis or respiratory alkalosis is corrected or controlled; ABG is returning to or have returned to normal range.
- The client remains free of signs and symptoms of respiratory acidosis or respiratory alkalosis.
- The client exhibits a patent airway and the breath sounds have improved.
- The client ambulates with little or no assistance and without breathlessness.
- Document compliance with prescribed drug therapy and medical regimen.

Intravenous Therapy

▶ INTRODUCTION

This unit discusses the basic classifications of intravenous solutions in terms of their osmolality and the various types of fluids for intravenous administration. The two chapters in this unit are Intravenous Administration and Total Parenteral Nutrition (TPN). Purposes for IV therapy include: (1) hydration to restore fluid loss (rehydrate) and improve renal output; (2) maintenance to meet daily fluid needs; (3) replacement for ongoing fluid losses; and (4) replacement of electrolyte losses.

Many of the solutions used for IV therapy are produced commercially to meet clients' needs associated with specific types of fluid, electrolyte, and acid-base imbalances. IV solutions are classified as being hypotonic, isotonic, or hypertonic. IV osmolality of a solution is determined by the concentration or the number of particles (osmols) suspended in the solution. The greater the number of particles in the solution, the higher the osmolality of the solution. Hypotonic (hypo-osmolar) solutions have less than 240 mOsm/L; isotonic (iso-osmolar) solutions have approximately 240–340 mOsm/L; and hypertonic (hyperosmolar) solutions have more than 340 mOsm/L. Table U4-1 lists IV solutions according to their osmolality and uses; e.g., hydrating solutions, replacement solutions, protein solutions, and plasma expanders.

▶ CRYSTALLOIDS

Commonly used crystalloid solutions include dextrose and water (D_5W), saline (NSS), and lactated Ringer's solutions. Isotonic solutions such as 5% dextrose and water (D_5W) have approximately 250 mOsm/L. A normal saline solution (0.9% NaCl or NSS) has 310 mOsm/L, and lactated Ringer's solution has approximately the same number of milliosmols. Hypotonic solutions include 0.33% NaCl (one-third normal saline)

Table U4-1

Selected Solutions Used in IV Therapy

Categories and Solutions	Tonicity (Osmolality)	Electrolytes (mEq/L)	Rationale
Hydrating Solutions			
0.45% NaCl [½ normal saline solution (NSS)]	Hypotonic	Na: 77, Cl: 77	Useful for establishing renal function. Not for replacement therapy.
Dextrose 2.5% in 0.45% saline	Isotonic	Calories: 85, Na: 77, Cl: 77	Helpful in establishing renal function.
Dextrose 5% in 0.2% saline	Isotonic	Calories: 170, Na: 38, Cl: 38	Useful for daily maintenance of body fluids when less Na and Cl are required.
Dextrose 5% in 0.33% saline	Hypertonic	Calories: 170, Na: 51, Cl: 51	Useful for daily maintenance of body fluids.
Dextrose 5% in 0.45% saline	Hypertonic	Calories: 170, Na: 77, Cl: 77	Useful for daily maintenance of body fluids and for treating fluid volume deficits.
Dextrose 5% in water (Dextrose 10% in water is occasionally used)	Isotonic	Calories: 170	Helpful in rehydration and elimination. May cause urinary sodium loss. Good vehicle for IV potassium.
Replacement Solutions			
Dextrose 5% in 0.9% NaCl [(normal saline solution NSS)]	Hypertonic	Calories: 170, Na: 154, Cl: 154	Replacement of fluid, sodium, chloride, and calories.
Lactated Ringer's	Isotonic	Na: 130, K: 4, Ca: 3, Cl: 109, lactate: 28	Resembles the electrolyte composition of normal blood serum/plasma. Potassium amount does not meet body's daily K requirement.
Dextrose 5% in lactated Ringer's	Hypertonic	Calories: 170, Na: 130, K: 4, Ca: 3, Cl: 109, lactate:28	Same contents as lactated Ringer's plus calories.
Ringer's solution	Isotonic	Na: 147, K: 4, Ca: 3, Cl: 154	Does not contain lactate, which may be harmful to clients who lack enzymes essential to metabolize lactic acid.
Normal saline solution (NSS)	Isotonic	Na: 154, Cl: 154	Restores ECF volume and replaces sodium and chloride deficits.
Hypertonic saline 3% NaCl	Hypertonic	Na: 513, Cl: 513	Helpful in hyponatremia. Helpful in eliminating intracellular fluid excess.

continues on the following page

D₅W - isotonic but dextrose is metabolized, it becomes hypotonic

Table U4-1

(Continued)

Categories and Solutions	Tonicity (Osmolality)	Electrolytes (mEq/L)	Rationale
Protein Solutions			
Aminosyn RF 5.2%	Hypertonic	Calories: 175, K: 5.4, amino acids	Provides protein and fluid for the body and promotes wound healing.
Aminosyn II 3.5% with dextrose 5%	Hypertonic	Calories: 345, Na: 18, amino acids	Provides protein, calories, and fluids. Helpful for the malnourished and for clients with hypoproteinemia. Not to be used in severe liver damage.
Plasma Expander			
Dextran 40 in normal saline or 5% dextrose⁻ in water	Isotonic		Colloidal solution used to increase plasma volume. Dextran 40 is a short-lived plasma volume expander (4 to 6 hours). Useful in early shock to correct hypovolemia, increase arterial blood pressure, improve pulse pressure and cardiac output. It improves microcirculation and increases small vessel perfusion. *Caution:* NOT to be used in severely dehydrated clients, in renal disease, thrombocytopenia, or clients who are actively hemorrhaging.

(handwritten annotations: "No! to severely dehydrated pts", "yes", "No!")

Compiled from Abbott Laboratories Wall Chart; "Guide to Fluid Therapy," 1981, Deerfield, IN: Travenol Laboratories, Inc.; *Fluid and Electrolyte Balance: Nursing Considerations* (3rd ed.), by N. M. Metheny, 1996, Philadelphia: Lippincott; *A Primer of Water, Electrolyte, and Acid-Base Syndromes* (8th ed.), by J. M. Brensilver and E. Goldberger, 1996, Philadelphia: F. A. Davis.

with 103 mOsm/L, and 0.45% NaCl (one-half normal saline) with 154 mOsm/L. *Although 5% dextrose and water is isotonic, it becomes a hypotonic solution as soon as the dextrose is metabolized in the body.* When 5% dextrose and water and without sodium chloride is used consistently over a period of time, the client is actually receiving a hypotonic solution, which can cause ICFVE or water intoxication. Hypertonic solu-

5gm dextrose in 100 mL

tions include 5% dextrose with 0.9% NaCl (NSS), which contains 560 mOsm/L, 5% dextrose in lactated Ringer's solution (525 mOsm/L), and 3% saline solution (810 mOsm/L).

Dextrose solutions for intravenous therapy are prepared in two strengths, 5% and 10%. Five percent dextrose means that there are 5 grams of dextrose in 100 mL of solution. Therefore, 1 L or 1000 mL of 5% dextrose contains 50 grams (50 g) of dextrose. One gram of dextrose is equivalent to 4 calories, thus 50 grams is equivalent to 200 calories. One liter of 5% dextrose and water does not supply many calories. Potassium that is administered intravenously must be diluted in a solution such as 5% dextrose and water. Potassium should *never* be given as a bolus injection because lethal cardiac dysrhythmias will result.

Normal saline solution (NSS or 0.9% NaCl) is isotonic and similar to plasma; however, it contains a slightly higher concentration of sodium chloride (Na = 154 mEq/L and Cl = 154 mEq/L). NSS is useful in replacing fluid and ECF electrolyte losses. It is considered a plasma volume expander. A hypertonic saline solution (3% NaCl) may be used in treating a client with severe hyponatremia; the serum sodium level is usually <115 mEq/L.

Lactated Ringer's solution is similar to plasma. It contains sodium, potassium, calcium chloride, and lactate (lactate is metabolized to bicarbonate). It is isotonic and frequently called a balanced electrolyte solution (BES). This solution is usually prescribed following trauma or surgery to replace "plasma-like" fluid. Lactated Ringer's and normal saline solutions can be used interchangeably for acute fluid replacement.

There are numerous commercially-prepared, balanced electrolyte solutions. Most of these IV solutions contain sodium, potassium, magnesium, chloride, and either acetate, lactate, or gluconate; some also contain calcium and phosphate. These solutions are prescribed for either maintenance needs or for replacement losses such as severe vomiting, burns, diabetic acidosis, or postoperative dehydration. Table U4-2 lists commercially-produced, balanced electrolyte solutions according to the companies that manufacture these products.

▶ COLLOIDS *Volume expanders*

Colloids are frequently called volume expanders or plasma expanders; they physiologically function like plasma proteins in the blood by maintaining oncotic pressure. Commonly used colloids include albumin, dextran, Plasmanate, and hetastarch (artificial blood substitute). Hypotension and allergic reactions can occur with their use.

Dextran is a colloidal solution that is used to expand the plasma volume. Dextran can affect clotting by coating the platelets and reducing their ability to clot. Dextran comes in two concentrations, dextran 40 and

Table U4-2

Commercially-Prepared Balanced Electrolyte Solutions

Solution	mEq/L Concentration
Abbott Solutions	
Normosol R	Na: 140; K: 5; Mg: 3; Cl: 98; Acetate: 27; Gluconate: 23
Normosol M	Na: 40; K: 13; Mg: 3; Cl: 40; Acetate: 16
Ionosol B	
(also in 5% dextrose)	Na: 57; K: 25; Mg: 5; Cl: 49; HPO$_4$: 7; lactate: 25
Ionosol MB	
(also in 5% dextrose)	Na: 25; K: 20; Mg: 3; Cl: 22; HPO$_4$: 3; lactate: 23
Baxter Solutions	
Plasma-Lyte 148	Na: 140; K: 5; Mg: 3; Cl: 98; Acetate: 27; Gluconate: 23
Plasma-Lyte R	Na: 140; K: 10; Ca: 5; Mg: 3; Cl: 103; Acetate: 47; lactate: 8
Plasma-Lyte M	Na: 40; K: 16; Ca: 5; Mg: 3; Cl: 40; Acetate: 12; lactate: 12
McGaw Solutions	
Isolyte E	Na: 140; K: 10; Ca: 5; Mg: 3; Cl: 103; Acetate: 49; Citrate: 8
Isolyte S	Na: 140; K: 5; Mg: 3; Cl: 98; Acetate: 27; Gluconate: 23
Isolyte R	Na: 40; K: 16; Ca: 5; Mg: 3; Cl: 40; Acetate: 24
Isolyte M	Na: 38; K: 35; Cl: 40; HPO$_4$: 15; Acetate: 20

Compiled from *Fluid and Electrolyte Balance: Nursing Considerations* (3rd ed.), by N. M. Metheny, 1996, Philadelphia: Lippincott; *A Primer of Water, Electrolyte, and Acid-Base Syndromes* (8th ed.), by J. M. Brensilver and E. Goldberger, 1996, Philadelphia: Davis.

Colloid: Albumin, Dextran [handwritten annotation]

dextran 70. Dextran 40 remains in the circulatory system for 6 hours and dextran 70 remains in circulation for 20 hours. Dextran 70 is infrequently used because it can cause severe dehydration and can affect blood typing and cross-matching. Dextran 40 is useful in correcting hypovolemia in early shock by increasing arterial blood pressure and increasing cardiac output; it also increases pulse pressure. Another purpose for dextran 40 is to improve microcirculation by reducing red blood cell aggregation in the capillaries.

The use of dextran 40 is contraindicated for clients having severe dehydration, renal disease, thrombocytopenia, or active hemorrhaging. In severe dehydration, dextran 40 increases dehydration by pulling more fluid from the cells and tissue spaces into the vascular space. If urine output is good, the vascular fluid is excreted. Both cellular and extracellular dehydration occur. However, if renal function is decreased, fluid hypervolemia might occur. If oliguria is due to hypovolemia, dextran 40 may improve urine output, but if renal damage is present, dextran 40 may cause renal failure. Dextran 40 tends to clot platelets and prolong bleeding time, so this solution is not indicated for a client with thrombocytopenia. Dextran 40 improves microcirculation, and during active bleeding, additional blood loss can occur from the capillaries if hemorrhage is prolonged.

Albumin concentrate is useful in restoring body protein. It is considered to be a plasma volume expander. Too much albumin or albumin administered too rapidly can cause fluid to be retained in the pulmonary vasculature. Plasmanate is a commercially-prepared protein product that is used instead of plasma and albumin to replace body protein.

▶ BLOOD AND BLOOD COMPONENTS

Blood and blood components are another type of intravenous therapy. Whole blood, plasma, and platelets can be administered intravenously. Fifty-five percent of whole blood is plasma. Various components of whole blood can be fractionated and transfused separately. These components include red blood cells (RBC or packed cells), plasma, platelets, white blood cells (WBC), albumin, and blood factors II, VII, VIII, IX, and X. Red blood cells, also known as packed cells, are composed of whole blood minus the plasma. A unit of RBC or packed cells is 250 mL. When RBC replacement is needed without an increase in fluid volume, a unit of RBC is often prescribed instead of whole blood.

The shelf life of refrigerated whole blood is 42 days. Red blood cells and plasma can be frozen to extend their shelf life to 10 years for red blood cells and 1 year for plasma. Platelets must be administered within 5 days after they have been extracted from whole blood. As whole blood ages, potassium leaves the red blood cells, thus increasing the serum potassium level. After 3 weeks of shelf life, serum potassium in the whole blood can increase to 20 mEq/L or greater. A client who has an elevated or a slightly elevated serum potassium level should not receive whole blood that has a long shelf life. This "old blood" could dangerously increase the client's serum potassium level.

The hematocrit measures the volume of red blood cells in proportion to the extracellular fluid. A rise or drop in the hematocrit can indicate a gain or loss of intravascular extracellular fluid. An increased concentration of red blood cells is known as hemoconcentration. A transfusion of whole blood or plasma decreases the hemoconcentration, thus lowering the hematocrit, increasing the blood pressure, and establishing renal flow. The treatment of choice to decrease osmolality is a transfusion of plasma or the administration of crystalloids.

1 unit = 250 mL

Intravenous Administration

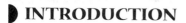

▶ INTRODUCTION

Concepts related to intravenous administration and therapy are presented in this chapter through the use of six subheadings: (1) basic purposes of IV therapy, (2) IV flow rate and calculation for IV infusion, (3) types of IV infusion devices for short-term IV therapy, (4) central venous catheters for long-term IV therapy, (5) assessment factors in IV therapy, and (6) possible complications resulting from IV administration. Client Management, including assessment, diagnoses, interventions, and evaluation/outcome summarize the important functions for the health professional.

▶ BASIC PURPOSES OF INTRAVENOUS THERAPY

Healthy persons normally do not require fluid and electrolyte therapy; however, certain illnesses and conditions compromise the body's ability to adapt to fluid changes. When a client cannot maintain this balance, IV therapy may be indicated. Persons requiring intravenous therapy may depend on intravenous therapy to meet daily maintenance needs for water, electrolytes, calories, vitamins, and other nutritional substances.

The five purposes of IV therapy are to: (1) provide maintenance requirements for fluids and electrolytes, (2) replace previous losses, (3) replace concurrent losses, (4) provide nutrition, and (5) provide a mechanism for the administration of medications and/or the transfusion of blood and blood components. Multiple electrolyte solutions are helpful in replacing previous and concurrent fluid losses. Fluid and electrolyte losses that occur from diarrhea, vomiting, and/or gastric suction are an example of concurrent losses. When a client is unable to meet his or her nutritional needs through oral intake, total parenteral nutrition (TPN) may be prescribed; TPN is discussed in Chapter 14. IV therapy is also used for administering medications and blood products. Sufficient kidney function is necessary while the client is receiving IV fluids and electrolyte therapy. Renal dysfunction may result in fluid overload and electrolyte imbalances.

Fluids and electrolytes for maintenance therapy should be ordered on a daily basis and administered over a period of 24 hours. If a client receives his or her full 24-hour maintenance parenteral therapy in 8 hours, two-thirds of the water and electrolytes are in excess of the body's current needs, and a large portion of the excess maintenance fluids is excreted.

Tolerance for sudden changes in water and electrolytes is limited for extremely ill clients following major surgery, elderly clients, small children, and infants. Rapid administration of replacement fluids that exceed a person's physiologic tolerance can cause hyponatremia, pulmonary edema, and other complications.

▶ IV FLOW RATE AND CALCULATIONS FOR INTRAVENOUS INFUSIONS

The desired amount of solution (mL) per day and the IV flow rate are generally calculated in relation to the type of therapy needed; e.g., maintenance, replacement with maintenance, or hydration. Urinary output needs to be reestablished before maintenance therapy is started. Table 13-1 outlines the three types of IV therapy, the amount of suggested IV solutions, and the suggested IV flow rate. The IV flow rate may need to be adjusted if the client is very ill, elderly, a small child, or infant. Today, many institutions use IV controllers or pumps to deliver IV fluids. The health professional needs to know how to calculate the flow rate and regulate the various types of infusion devices.

Table 13-1

Types of IV Therapy

Type of Therapy	Amount of Solution Desired (mL)	Rate of Flow
Maintenance therapy	1500–2000	62–83 mL/h or 1–1.5 mL/min if given over 24 h
Replacement with maintenance therapy	2000–3000	83–125 mL/h or 1.5–2 mL/min (depends on individual)
Hydration therapy	1000–3000	60–120 mL/h or 1–2 mL/min

Note: These guidelines may be adapted to individual circumstances. The health care provider orders the 24-h requirements and the health professional computes 1-h requirements from this. The amount of solution to be administered and the rate of flow can vary greatly with the very sick, the elderly, the small child, the infant, and the postsurgical client.

Table 13-2

Intravenous Sets

Drops (gtt) Per Milliliter

Macrodrip Sets	Microdrip Sets
10 gtt/mL	60 gtt/mL
15 gtt/mL	
20 gtt/mL	

The prescribed order for IV therapy includes the type of fluid for infusion and the amount to be administered in a specified period of time. The health professional must compute the number of milliliters per hour (mL/h) and then calculate the drops per minute for the infusion. Electronic infusion pumps are frequently used to administer IV solutions and are usually regulated to deliver milliliters per hour.

When using IV infusion sets for IV therapy administration, first check the drop factor or drip rate that is printed on the manufacturer's box or package. The number of drops per milliliter (gtt/mL) varies with each manufacturer. Drop factors range from 10–20 gtt/mL for the macrodrip chambers and 60 gtt/mL for microdrip chambers. Table 13-2 lists the drop factors according to macrodrip sets and microdrip sets.

There are two methods used to calculate IV flow rate (gtt/minute):

Two-Step Method:

a. Amount of fluid ÷ hours to administer = mL/h

b. $\dfrac{\text{mLh} \times \text{gtt/mL (IV set)}}{60 \text{ min}}$ = gtt/min

One-Step Method:

$\dfrac{\text{Amount of fluid} \times \text{gtt/mL (IV set)}}{\text{Hours to administer} \times \text{Minutes per hour (60)}}$ = gtt/min

Example:
Order: 2000 mL of 5% dextrose in 0.45% NaCl (one-half normal saline solution) and 1000 mL of D$_5$W to run over 24 hours. The drop factor on the manufacturer's box is 10 gtt/mL. Using the two-step method, the client should receive 125 mL/h and 21 gtt/min.

Using the two-step method:

a. 3000 mL ÷ 24 h = 125 mL/h

b. $\dfrac{125 \text{ mL/h} \times 10 \text{ gtt/mL (IV set)}}{60 \text{ min (1 hr)}}$ = $\dfrac{1250}{60}$ = 21 gtt/min

Using the one-step method:

$\dfrac{3000 \text{ ml} \times 10 \text{ gtt/mL}}{24 \text{ h} \times 60 \text{ min}}$ = $\dfrac{30000}{1440}$ = 20.8 (21 gtt/min)

If the health professional uses an electronic IV infusion pump or controller, the volume per hour must be calculated (in this case 125 mL/h) and entered on the pump.

▶ TYPES OF IV INFUSION DEVICES FOR SHORT-TERM IV THERAPY

There are three common types of infusion devices for routine short-term IV therapy: the butterfly (steel needle), the over-needle catheter, and the inside-needle catheter. The winged-tip, or butterfly, set consists of a wing-tip needle with a steel cannula, plastic or rubber wings, and a plastic catheter or hub. The needle is $\frac{1}{2}$ to $1\frac{1}{2}$ inches long with needle gauges of 16 to 26. The infusion needle and clear tubing are bonded into a single unit.

Advantages of the butterfly infusion set are that it is a one-piece apparatus, has a short beveled needle, and is easy to tape securely. The butterfly reduces the risk of secondary puncture and infiltration on puncture. Disadvantages of this IV apparatus are that the butterfly should be used only for very short-term IV therapy (in many cases, less than 2 hours). The butterfly method is commonly used in children and the elderly whose veins are likely to be small or fragile.

The second type of commonly used IV device is the over-needle catheter (ONC). The bevel of the needle extends beyond the catheter, which is $1\frac{1}{4}$ to 8 inches in length. The needle is available in gauges of 12 to 24. With its short, large cannula, the ONC is preferable for rapid IV infusion and is more comfortable for the client. Catheters used in ONCs and INCs are constructed of silicone, Teflon, polyvinyl chloride, or polyethylene.

The third type of IV device is the inside-needle catheter (INC), which is constructed exactly the opposite of the ONC. Needle length is $1\frac{1}{2}$ to 3 inches with a catheter length of 8 to 25 inches. The catheter is available in gauges of 2 to 24. The INC set comes with a catheter sleeve guard that must be secured over the needle bevel to prevent severing the catheter. With its longer, narrower catheter, the INC is preferred when vein catheterization is necessary for prolonged infusions.

▶ CENTRAL VENOUS CATHETERS AND LONG-TERM IV THERAPY

Central venous catheters are another type of IV device. These catheters are radiopaque and may have a single, double, or triple lumen. Since the insertion of a central venous catheter presents critical risks, its insertion is followed by an x-ray to confirm the position and tip placement of the catheter.

Four common reasons for using a central venous catheter are: (1) to measure the central venous pressure, (2) for infusion of TPN, (3) for infusion of multiple IV fluids and/or medications, and (4) to infuse chemotherapeutic or irritating medications. Hickman, Groshong, and Cook are examples of central venous catheters that must be inserted in the operating room. The implantable vascular access device (IVAD) is another example of a central venous line that must be surgically inserted.

For clients without adequate peripheral sites and for those requiring long-term IV therapy, a central venous site is the optimal choice. Central venous sites are the superior vena cava and the inferior vena cava. The superior vena cava is accessed from the internal jugular vein and the right or left subclavian vein, whereas the inferior vena cava is accessed from the femoral vein. Figure 13-1 presents the central venous access sites. The catheter may be a single or multilumen. A peripherally inserted central catheter (PICC) line is used for long-term IV therapy (2 weeks to 1 year) and is frequently used in home care settings for clients who require IV therapy. The PICC line is inserted into the antecubital vein. A specifically trained or certified PICC insertion health professional inserts the catheter and an x-ray is taken to confirm accurate placement. Guidelines for flushing solutions and volume are presented in Table 13-3.

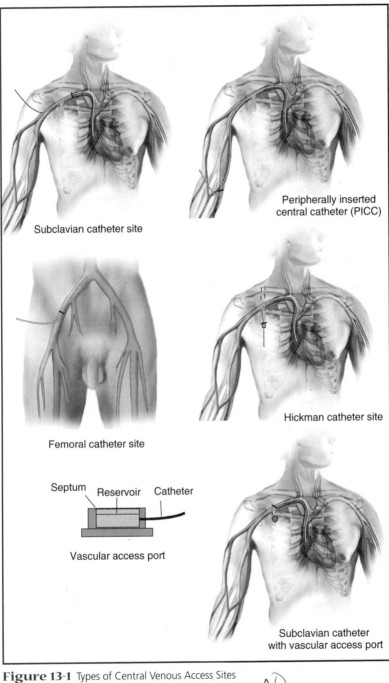

Figure 13-1 Types of Central Venous Access Sites

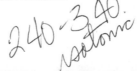

Table 13-3

Venous Access Devices: Flushing Guidelines

Type	Length (inches)	Flush Solution	Volume (mL)	Frequency
Peripheral Central Venous	1–2	Normal saline	1–3	After each use or q8h
Single lumen	8	Heparinized saline	1	After each use or q8h
Multilumen	8	Heparinized saline	1 port	After each use or q8h
External-tunneled Hickman, Cook, or Groshong	35	Heparinized saline	2–5	After each use or q8h
Peripherally inserted central catheter (PICC)	20	Normal saline	3–5	After each use or q12h
Implanted vascular access device	35	Heparinized saline	3–5	After each use; q5–7d when not in use

From *Clinical Calculations* (3rd ed.), by J. L. Kee and S. M. Marshall, 1995, Philadelphia: Saunders.

Complications that may occur with insertion of a central venous line into the subclavian and jugular veins are pneumothorax, hemorrhage, air embolism, thrombus dislodgement, and cardiac dysrhythmias. Long-term complications such as hemorrhage, phlebitis, air embolism, thrombus formation, infection, dislodgement, cardiac dysrhythmias, and circulatory impairment might occur with central venous lines.

▶ ASSESSMENT FACTORS IN INTRAVENOUS THERAPY

The IV solutions and devices are selected by the health professional. He or she must know and understand the various solutions, needles, catheters, tubings, IV sites, flow rate, positioning, and taping IV tubing in order to accurately assess, initiate, and monitor infusions. Table 13-4 provides the assessment factors, interventions, and rationale related to IV therapy.

Intravenous solutions with <240 mOsm are considered hypotonic. If a hypotonic solution is used continuously, ICFVE or water intoxication results. Five percent dextrose and water is an example of an isotonic solution that converts to a hypotonic solution when used continuously. Constant use of hyperosmolar solutions may cause dehydration.

Table 13-4

Assessment Factors in IV Therapy

Assessment	Interventions	Rationale
Types of IV Solutions	Note the types of IV fluid ordered: hypotonic, isotonic, or hypertonic solutions.	An excessive use of hypotonic solutions can cause a fluid volume excess. Excessive use of hypertonic solutions may cause a fluid volume deficit. An isotonic solution has 240–340 mOsm/L; less than 240 is hypo-osmolar, and greater than 340 is hyperosmolar.
	Report extended use of continuous IVs of dextrose in water.	Dextrose 5% in water administered continuously becomes a hypotonic solution. Dextrose is metabolized rapidly and the remaining water decreases the serum osmolality. Alternate use of D/W with D/NSS (saline) to prevent this complication.
	Observe for signs and symptoms of fluid volume deficit, i.e., dry mucous membranes, poor skin turgor, and increased pulse and respiration rates, when using hyperosmolar solutions. Creatinine/BUN ratio, 1:10/20; hemoconcentration, 1:20 or greater.	Continuous use of hyperosmolar solutions pulls fluid from intracellular compartments to the extracellular compartments. The fluid is excreted by the kidneys. Poor kidney function causes fluid retention, increasing the risk for a fluid volume excess.
Intravenous Tubing and Bag	Inspect IV bags for leaks by gently squeezing.	Microorganisms can enter IV bags through small leak sites, contaminating the fluid.
	Check drop size on the equipment box. Use IV tubing with macrodrip chamber (10–20 gtt/mL) for administering IV fluids at a rate of 50 mL/h or greater.	Use of a microdrip chamber (IV tubing) for fluids that are ordered to run at a rate greater than 50 mL/h is too slow and inaccurate.

continues on the following page

Table 13-4

(Continued)

Assessment	Interventions	Rationale
	Use microdrip chamber (60 gtt/mL) for administering IV fluids at a rate under 50 mL/h.	Infusion pumps increase the accuracy and decrease the risks associated with IV fluids that are to run for 12–24 h and meet specific client fluid needs.
	Change IV tubing every 24–48 h at time of new hanging.	Studies have shown that IV tubing left hanging for 48 h is free of bacteria when proper aseptic technique is used.
	New IV containers are hung according to agency policy.	An IV bag should not be used for longer than 24 h. If the order is for KVO (keep vein open), a 250–500-mL container with a microdrip chamber set is suggested.
Needles and IV Catheters (cannulas)	Recognize the types of IV needles and catheters used for IV fluids: Straight needles Scalp vein needles/ butterfly (steel) needles Heparin lock Over-needle-catheter (ONC) Inside-needle-catheter (INC)	Needles (straight and scalp vein) are used for short-term IV therapy and for clients with autoimmune problems. Catheters made of silicone and Teflon are less irritating than polyvinylchloride and polyethylene catheters.
	Change IV site every 2–3 days according to agency policy. Check the ONC for placement and function.	Needles and catheters in longer than 72 h increase the risk of phlebitis. There are many types of ONCs, i.e., Angiocath, A-Cath, Vicra Quik-Cath, etc. Catheter length can be 1–3 inches. Care should be taken to avoid severing the catheter with the needle tip.

continues on the following page

Table 13-4

(Continued)

Assessment	Interventions	Rationale
	Check for fluid leaks at the insertion site after the insertion of an INC.	An INC is used for central venous pressure monitoring, TPN (hyperalimentation), etc. It is frequently inserted in large veins, i.e., subclavian vein, internal jugular or femoral vein. Leaks result from needle punctures that are larger than the catheter.
Injection Site	Insert needle or catheter in the hand or the distal veins of the arm. Use the antecubital fossa (elbow) site last.	The upper extremity is preferred for the infusion site, since the occurrence of phlebitis and thrombosis in the upper extremities is not as prevalent as it is in the lower extremities.
	Avoid using the leg veins if possible.	Circulation in the leg veins is reduced and thrombus formation can occur.
	Avoid using limbs affected by a stroke or mastectomy for IV sites.	Circulation is usually decreased in affected extremities.
	Apply arm board and/or soft restraints to the extremity with the IV when the client is restless or confused.	Prevention of extremity movement with an IV decreases the chance of dislodging the needle and phlebitis.
Flow Rate and Irrigation	Check types of solutions clients are receiving.	Knowledge of tonicity (osmolality) of fluids aids in determining rate of flow. Rate of hypertonic solutions should be slower than isotonic solutions.
	Observe drip chamber and regulate accordingly.	Regulation of IV fluids is important to prevent overhydration, i.e., cough, dyspnea, neck vein engorgement, and chest rales. Do not play "catch-up" with IV fluids.

continues on the following page

Table 13-4

(Continued)

Assessment	Interventions	Rationale
	Regulate KVO (keep vein open) rate to run 10–20 mL/h or according to agency policy, or use an infusion pump.	KVO IVs should run approximately 10–20 mL/h.
	Label IV bag for milliliters (mL) to be received per hour. Check rate of flow every 30 min to 1 h with hypertonic and toxic solutions and every hour with isotonic solutions.	Hypertonic solutions administered rapidly can cause cellular dehydration and, if the kidneys are properly functioning, vascular dehydration. Hypertonic fluids act as an osmotic diuretic and can cause diuresis; when administered rapidly, speed shock can occur; and if extravasation occurs, necrotic tissue can result.
	Restore IV flow if stopped by opening flow clamp, milking the tubing, raising the height of IV bag, or repositioning the extremity.	If IV flow has stopped and does not start by opening clamp, milking tubing, raising the bag, or repositioning extremity, then the IV catheter should be removed. Irrigating IV catheters is prohibited in some institutions and should never be attempted with clotted lines. Forceful irrigation can dislodge clot(s) and cause the movement of an embolus to the lungs.
Position of IV Line	Position and tape IV tubing to prevent kinking.	Kinking of the tubing may cause the IV to be discontinued and to be restarted at a different site.
	Hang IV bag 2½–3 feet above client's infusion site.	The higher the IV bag, the faster the gravity flow rate. If the IV bag is too low, IV fluids may stop due to an insufficient gravity pull.

If IV fluids are to run at less than 50 mL per hour for 12 hours, IV tubing with a microdrip chamber is the best choice. IV tubing should be changed every 24 to 48 hours, and the IV container (bag) should not hang for longer than 24 hours. Needles and IV catheters should be changed at least every 3 days. The body areas preferred for the insertion of peripheral IV devices are hand veins and distal arm veins. The problem with the use of ONCs is severing of the catheter with the needle tip, and the problem with INCs is that a leak can occur at the infusion insertion site. IV fluids running too fast can cause overhydration.

▶ POSSIBLE COMPLICATIONS RESULTING FROM IV THERAPY

Numerous complications may result from the use of intravenous therapy. Infiltration, phlebitis, hematoma, and infections are common problems associated with IV infusions. Other serious problems include speed shock, air embolus, pulmonary embolus, and pulmonary edema. Speed shock occurs when drugs in solution are given too rapidly. It increases the drug concentration in the body and produces shocklike symptoms. An air embolus can be fatal when more than 50 mL of air is injected into the vein. Pulmonary embolus results when a thrombus in the peripheral veins becomes an embolus and travels to the lungs. This may occur when a clotted IV needle or catheter is irrigated forcefully, or when the lower extremities are used for administering IV fluids. Restlessness, chest pain, cough, dyspnea, and tachycardia are clinical signs and symptoms of a pulmonary embolus. Table 13-5 lists problems and complications that may occur from IV administration of fluids and medications.

▶ CLIENT MANAGEMENT

Assessment

- Check the prescribed IV solutions to ensure that the prescribed solutions are not all hypotonic or hypertonic. When 3000 mL of 5% dextrose in water is administered daily, this solution becomes hypotonic, and the dextrose is metabolized in the body, leaving water.

- Determine which IV tubing with drip chamber should be used. This is generally determined according to how long the IV fluids are to run. If the 1000 mL is to run 8 hours or more, the macrodrip chamber tubing should be selected.

Table 13-5

Possible Complications Resulting from IV Administration

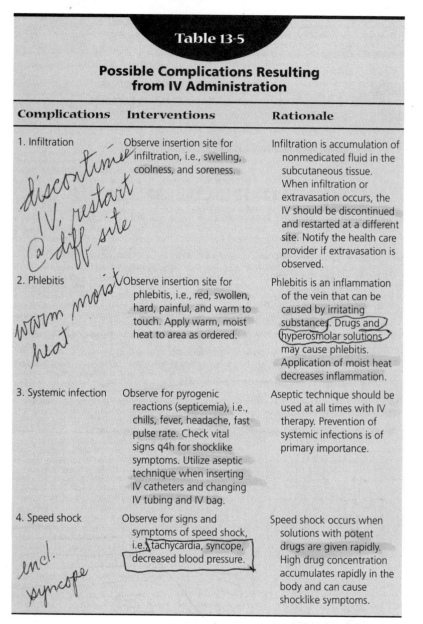

Complications	Interventions	Rationale
1. Infiltration	Observe insertion site for infiltration, i.e., swelling, coolness, and soreness.	Infiltration is accumulation of nonmedicated fluid in the subcutaneous tissue. When infiltration or extravasation occurs, the IV should be discontinued and restarted at a different site. Notify the health care provider if extravasation is observed.
2. Phlebitis	Observe insertion site for phlebitis, i.e., red, swollen, hard, painful, and warm to touch. Apply warm, moist heat to area as ordered.	Phlebitis is an inflammation of the vein that can be caused by irritating substances. Drugs and hyperosmolar solutions may cause phlebitis. Application of moist heat decreases inflammation.
3. Systemic infection	Observe for pyrogenic reactions (septicemia), i.e., chills, fever, headache, fast pulse rate. Check vital signs q4h for shocklike symptoms. Utilize aseptic technique when inserting IV catheters and changing IV tubing and IV bag.	Aseptic technique should be used at all times with IV therapy. Prevention of systemic infections is of primary importance.
4. Speed shock	Observe for signs and symptoms of speed shock, i.e., tachycardia, syncope, decreased blood pressure.	Speed shock occurs when solutions with potent drugs are given rapidly. High drug concentration accumulates rapidly in the body and can cause shocklike symptoms.

Handwritten annotations: "discontinue IV, restart @ diff. site" (next to Infiltration); "warm moist heat" (next to Phlebitis); "incl. syncope" (next to Speed shock).

continues on the following page

Table 13-5

(Continued)

Complications	Interventions	Rationale
5. Air embolism	Remove air from tubing to prevent air embolism.	Air can be removed from tubing by (1) inserting a needle with syringe into side arm of tubing set and withdrawing the air and (2) using a pen or pencil on tubing, distal to the air, and rolling tubing until air is displaced into the drip chamber.
	Observe for signs and symptoms of air embolism. These include pallor, dyspnea, cough, syncope, tachycardia, decreased blood pressure.	Air embolism occurs when air inadvertently enters the vascular system. Injection of more than 50 mL of air can be fatal. It occurs more frequently in the central veins, and symptoms usually appear within 5 min.
	Immediately place client on left side in Trendelenburg position.	Air is trapped in the right atrium, which prevents it from going to the lungs.
6. Pulmonary embolism	Report signs and symptoms of pulmonary embolism, i.e., restlessness, chest pain, cough, dyspnea, tachycardia.	Thrombus originating in the peripheral vein becomes an embolus and can lodge in a pulmonary vessel.
	Administer oxygen, analgesics, anticoagulants, and IV fluids as ordered.	Preventive measures should be taken, such as *never* forcefully irrigating an IV catheter to reestablish flow and avoiding the use of veins in the lower extremities.

[handwritten annotations: ↑ pallor, ↓ BP, ↑ HR; + Chest pn; PE; Avoid LE; ⊘ forceful irrigation]

continues on the following page

Table 13-5

(Continued)

Complications	Interventions	Rationale
7. Pulmonary edema	Auscultate lungs for crackles (rales). Check neck veins for engorgement. Decrease IV flow rate.	IV fluids administered too rapidly or in large amounts can cause overhydration. Excess fluids accumulate in the lungs.
8. "Runaway" IV fluids	Monitor IV fluid every hour even if on an electronic infusion pump (EIP). Check EIP flow rate and alarm set.	Control clamp on IV tubing is opened. Alarm was not set properly on EIP.
9. Hematoma	Observe for hematoma with unsuccessful attempts to start IV therapy. Apply ice pack immediately, then warm compresses after 1 hour.	Hematoma (blood tumor) is a raised ecchymosed area. Ice stops bleeding into the tissue. Warm compresses cause vasodilation and improve blood flow and healing.
Additives to IV Fluids	Recognize the untoward reactions of drugs in IV fluids: potassium, Levophed, low-pH drugs, vitamins, antibiotics, antineoplastic drugs.	Potassium, antineoplastic drugs, and Levophed irritate the blood vessels and body tissue. Phlebitis is common with these drugs; and if infiltration occurs, sloughing of tissues may result. Vitamins and antibiotics should not be mixed together. They are incompatible. Always check compatibility charts before adding medications to IV fluids.
	Stay with the client 10–15 min when the client is receiving drugs that are classified as a possible cause of anaphylaxis.	Allergic reactions often occur within the first 15 min when drugs are administered by IV.

continues on the following page

Table 13-5

(Continued)

Complications	Interventions	Rationale
	Inject drugs into IV container and invert several times before administering.	Equal drug distribution throughout the solution ensures proper dilution. *Do not* add drugs, i.e., potassium, into the IV bag while it is being administered unless the IV is temporarily stopped and the bag is inverted several times to promote equal distribution.
Intake and Output	Check urine output every 4–8 h. If a critically ill client is receiving potassium, urine output should be checked every hour.	If renal function is poor, overhydration can occur when excessive or continuous IV fluids are given. Potassium is excreted by the kidneys; thus, a decreased urine output can result in hyperkalemia.

- Select and observe infusion sites carefully. To reduce the risk of phlebitis and dislodged thrombus, the upper extremities are preferred infusion sites.
- Calculate flow rates and regulate the IV solutions. Patency of the IV system and regulation of the flow rate are essential.
- Assess for problems and complications of IV infusion.

Diagnoses

- *Fluid Volume Excess,* related to runaway IV or volume infusion too great for client's physical condition.
- *Risk for Fluid Volume Deficit,* related to inadequate fluid intake.

- *Risk for Infection,* related to contaminated IV fluid, contaminated equipment, or a break in aseptic technique.
- *Knowledge Deficit,* related to a lack of familiarity with IV therapy or infusion devices.

Interventions

- Monitor the rate of IV flow. Avoid fluid overload from IV solutions that run too fast. Pulmonary edema can result. IV solutions that run too slowly can cause an inadequate fluid intake.
- Monitor vital signs and chest sounds for signs of fluid overload; these include tachycardia, dyspnea, chest rales, and vein engorgements.
- Use aseptic technique when inserting an infusion device, changing IV tubing, changing IV bags, and changing site dressings. A break in the system provides the potential for bacterial invasion.
- Change peripheral IV site, IV tubing, and dressing sites according to the agency's policy.
- Check frequently for fluid leaks from IV site and tubing, and for pain, redness, and swelling at the site.
- Monitor urine output. Decreased urinary output may be an indication of fluid overload or dehydration.
- Monitor laboratory results, particularly serum electrolytes, BUN, serum creatinine, hematocrit, and hemoglobin. These results can indicate overhydration, dehydration, and/or electrolyte imbalances.

Evaluation/Outcome

- Evaluate the effects of intravenous therapy to replace fluid and electrolyte losses, to meet concurrent fluid losses, and maintain fluid balance.
- Evaluate the tonicity of the prescribed daily IV fluids to avoid constant use of either hypotonic or hypertonic solutions.
- The client remains free of problems and complications, such as phlebitis, infiltration, fluid overload, air embolus, and pulmonary embolus, related to IV therapy.

Total Parenteral Nutrition (TPN)

[handwritten annotations: Central Venous administration, R subclavian vein, IJ]

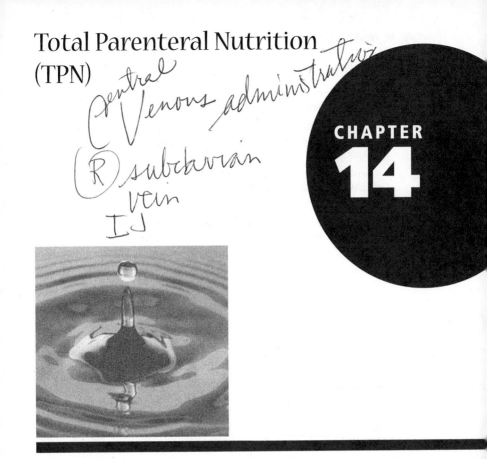

▶ INTRODUCTION

Total parenteral nutrition (TPN), sometimes referred to as hyperalimentation, is the infusion of amino acids, hypertonic glucose, and additives such as vitamins, electrolytes, minerals, and trace elements. TPN can meet a client's total nutritional needs and is commonly used for clients whose caloric intake is insufficient. This method of nutrition is recommended for those who need nutritional support for a long period of time and cannot tolerate enteral feedings. Administering a high concentration of glucose solutions in peripheral veins can cause phlebitis at the infusion site; therefore, central vein administration is used for TPN. Central veins such as the right subclavian vein and the internal jugular vein can accommodate a high volume of hypertonic solutions because of their size and ability to dilute the infused fluid.

▶ ETIOLOGY   *Restores (+) nitrogen balance*

Candidates for TPN include clients: with severe burns who are in negative nitrogen balance; who cannot take enteral feedings; with severe debilitating diseases (cancer, AIDS); with gastrointestinal disorders such as ulcerative colitis, gastrointestinal fistulas, and other GI conditions in which the GI tract cannot consume enteral feedings.

For clients who are unable to tolerate oral or gastric feeding and suffer from severe malnutrition, TPN helps to restore a positive nitrogen balance. Following a major bowel resection, the absorptive area of the intestines is reduced; TPN aids in providing adequate nutrients. The benefit TPN provides clients with a gastrointestinal fistula is to allow the intestine to rest while providing nutrients. Table 14-1 lists indications for TPN.

▶ TPN SOLUTIONS

The typical TPN solution for 1 L or 1000 mL contains 25% dextrose mixed in a commercially-prepared protein (amino acid) source. Vitamins and electrolytes are added prior to administration. Electrolytes are frequently added immediately before the infusion according to the client's serum electrolyte levels. Frequently, the pharmacy department prepares these solutions using aseptic technique under a laminar airflow hood according to the prescribed order. Dextrose (glucose) is the choice carbohydrate for TPN because it can be metabolized by all tissues. The protein source for TPN is crystalline amino acids. Intravenous fat emulsions may also be given through an extra line. Clients with diabetes mellitus may need a higher percentage of fat emulsion to prevent hyperglycemia. Standard TPN solutions contain dextrose, amino acids, sodium, potassium (added later), magnesium, calcium, chloride, phosphate, acetate, vitamins (added later), and trace elements. Other additives may be included according to individual needs.

Daily TPN solutions can be administered through a Hickman catheter or PICC line as a continuous infusion or intermittent infusion that runs for approximately 12 hours. By having a 12-hour TPN infusion time, the client is free the remaining 12 hours for normal activities, such as work, school, or play. Today, many clients receive the 12-hour method of infusion in the home. A support system is usually available for client's needs and questions.

Usually 1 L of solution is ordered for the first 24 hours when initiating TPN therapy. This allows the pancreas to accommodate the increased glucose concentration of the solution. Additional daily increases of 500 to 1000 mL per day are ordered until the desired daily volume is reached. A usual maintenance volume of $2\frac{1}{2}$ to 3 liters of the hypertonic TPN so-

Table 14-1

Indications for TPN (Hyperalimentation)

Indications	Rationale
Oral or nasogastric feedings are contraindicated or not tolerated	Long-term use of IV glucose solutions can cause protein wasting. TPN maintains a positive nitrogen balance.
Severe malnutrition	Malnutrition can cause severe protein loss and wasting syndrome. Negative nitrogen (protein) balance occurs. TPN restores positive nitrogen balance.
Malabsorption syndrome	The inability to absorb nutrients in the small intestine requires nutrients to be offered intravenously.
Dysphagia	Difficulty in masticating and swallowing due to pharyngeal radiation treatment prevents clients from breaking down food sufficiently for digestion.
Gastrointestinal fistula	Fistulas promote protein losses. TPN allows the intestine to rest and decreases gall bladder, pancreas, and small intestine secretions.
Major bowel resection and ulcerative colitis	These disorders reduce the absorptive area of the small intestine. TPN increases the intestine's ability to absorb nutrients more quickly than oral feedings and it permits the bowel to rest.
Extensive surgical trauma and stress	Extensive surgery requires 3500–5000 calories a day to maintain protein balance. TPN lowers the chance for infection and provides a positive nitrogen balance to aid in wound healing. TPN before surgery improves the nutritional status so that the client can withstand surgery and its stresses.
Extensive burns	Extensive burns require 7500–10,000 calories daily. TPN improves wound healing and formation of granulation tissue and promotes successful skin grafting.
Metastatic cancer or AIDS with anorexia and weight loss	Clients with wasting syndrome and debilitating diseases, such as cancer or AIDS, frequently are in negative nitrogen balance. TPN restores protein balance and tissue synthesis.

lution is administered over 24 hours. A continuous infusion rate prevents fluctuations in blood glucose levels. If blood sugar levels are under control, a 12-hour TPN method may be used.

Medications should not be administered in TPN solutions. A multilumen central venous catheter or an additional peripheral site must be used if the client requires IV fluids, blood products, and/or IV medications.

▶ ELECTROLYTE AND GLUCOSE IMBALANCES ASSOCIATED WITH TPN

Because of high glucose concentration, potassium shifts from the extracellular fluid sites to the cells (ICF). Increased potassium is needed in the TPN solutions, otherwise the client's potassium level begins to fall after 8–12 hours of TPN therapy. Hypokalemia may result from clients receiving insulin to manage hyperglycemia. Insulin moves potassium back into the cells. The client should generally receive 60 to 90 mEq of potassium per day in the TPN solutions (in some cases, more potassium per day is added to the solutions). Hyperkalemia may result from decreased renal function, systemic sepsis, or tissue necrosis. Serum potassium levels and urine output need to be closely monitored while the client is receiving potassium.

Hypophosphatemia (decreased serum phosphorus level) is a common problem associated with TPN. Increased glucose concentration in TPN solutions moves phosphate back into the cells. During TPN therapy, protein synthesis promotes the shift of phosphates back into the cells.

Hypomagnesemia does not occur as frequently as hypokalemia and hypophosphatemia; however, it can occur in clients who are severely malnourished, have excessive loss of intestinal secretions, have a long-term alcoholic problem, or are receiving daily magnesium-wasting diuretics.

Hyponatremia and hypocalcemia are not as common as hypokalemia and hypophosphatemia. A decreased serum sodium level may result from syndrome of inappropriate antidiuretic hormone (SIADH) or from excessive fluid intake. Hypocalcemia usually results from a decrease in albumin levels associated with malnutrition. Hypercalcemia may occur during long-term TPN therapy. This results from calcium loss from the bone. Table 14-2 lists the types of electrolyte and glucose imbalances, amount of daily electrolyte requirement, and causes of the imbalance.

Hyperglycemia is a problem related to the high glucose concentration of TPN solutions. Excess blood glucose levels occur more frequently during early TPN therapy. Other causes include rapidly infused glucose solutions, stress, and illness. TPN is primarily started with one liter of solution for the first day and then the volume of solution is increased to meet the client's needs.

▶ COMPLICATIONS RELATED TO TPN

Major complications that can result from TPN therapy are air embolus, phlebitis, thrombus, infection, hyperglycemia or hypoglycemia, and fluid overload. TPN is an excellent medium for the growth of organisms, bacteria, and yeast. Strict asepsis is necessary when IV tubing and dressings are changed. Most hospitals have a procedure for changing dressings in which strict aseptic technique, i.e., gloves, masks, and antibiotic ointment, is mandated.

Table 14-2

Electrolyte and Glucose Imbalances Related to TPN

Imbalances	Suggested Replacement	Causes
Electrolytes		
Hypokalemia	60–90 mEq/d	High blood glucose levels Insulin
Hyperkalemia		Decreased renal function Systemic sepsis Tissue necrosis
Hypophosphatemia	15–45 mEq/d	High blood glucose levels Protein synthesis
Hypomagnesemia	4–40 mEq/d	Severely malnourished Excessive loss of intestinal secretions Chronic alcohol problem
Hyponatremia	30–50 mEq/L	SIADH Excessive fluid intake
Hypocalcemia	5–10 mEq/L	Decreased albumin levels Malnourishment
Glucose		
Hyperglycemia	25% dextrose/L	Rapidly administered TPN solutions Stress Illness

When IV tubing is changed at the central venous catheter site, the client must lie flat and perform the Valsalva maneuver (take a breath, hold it, and bear down) to prevent air from being sucked into the circulation. The Valsalva maneuver increases intrathoracic pressure.

Increased blood glucose (hyperglycemia) occurs as a result of rapid infusion of the hypertonic dextrose solution used in TPN. An elevated blood glucose level may occur during early TPN until the pancreas adjusts to the hyperglycemic load. Regular insulin, either in the IV solution or by subcutaneous injection, may be required to prevent or control hyperglycemia. Other complications that can occur include hypoglycemia from abruptly discontinuing hyperosmolar dextrose solutions, fluid volume excess from the infusion of an excessive volume of fluid, or a fluid shift from intracellular to extracellular compartments. Table 14-3 lists the five major complications associated with TPN therapy (hyperalimentation), their related causes, symptoms, and corresponding interventions.

Table 14-3

Complications of TPN

Complications	Causes	Symptoms	Interventions
Air embolism	IV tubing disconnected Catheter not clamped Injection port fell off Improper changing of IV tubing (no Valsalva procedure)	Coughing Shortness of breath Chest pain Cyanosis	Clamp catheter Client must lie on left side with head down Check vital signs (VS) Notify health care provider
Infection	Poor aseptic technique when catheter inserted Contamination when changing tubing Contamination when solution mixed Contamination when dressing changed	Temperature above 100° (37.7°C) Pulse increased Chills Sweating Redness, swelling, drainage at insertion site Pain in neck, arm, or shoulder Lethargy Urine: glycosuria Bacteria Yeast growth	Notify health care provider Change dressing every 24–48 h according to agency policy Change solution every 24 h Change tubing every 24 h according to agency policy Check VS every 4 h
Hyperglycemia	Fluids rapidly infused Insufficient insulin coverage Infection	Nausea Weakness Thirst Headache Blood glucose elevated	Monitor blood glucose Notify health care provider Decrease infusion rate Regular insulin as required Monitor blood glucose every 4 h and prn

continues on the following page

Table 14-3

(Continued)

Complications	Causes	Symptoms	Interventions
Hypoglycemia	Fluids abruptly discontinued Too much insulin infused	Nausea Pallor Cold, clammy Increased pulse rate Shaky feeling Headache Blurred vision	Notify health care provider Increase infusion rate with NO insulin, as per order or hospital policy *or* Orange juice with 2 teaspoons of sugar if client can tolerate fluids *or* Glucose IV, as per order or hospital policy *or* Glucagon, as per order or hospital policy
Fluid overload (hypervolemia)	Increased rate of IV infusions Fluid shift from cellular to vascular due to hyperosmolar solutions	Cough Dyspnea Neck vein engorgement Chest rales Weight gain	Check VS every 4 h Weigh daily Monitor intake and output Check neck veins for engorgement Check chest sounds Monitor electrolytes Monitor BUN and creatinine

Source: Adapted from "Helping Your Client Settle in with TPN" by L. Wilhelm, 1985, *Nursing 85*, *15*(4), p. 63. Copyright 1985 by Springhouse Corporation. Reprinted with permission.

Hypertonic dextrose in a protein hydrolysate solution promotes yeast and bacteria growth. It has been reported that these organisms do not grow as rapidly in a crystalline amino acid solution as they do in protein hydrolysate solution. Many of the TPN solutions contain a crystalline amino acid solution, not a protein hydrolysate solution.

▶ CLIENT MANAGEMENT

Assessment

- Check TPN solutions, infusion site, and IV line. TPN lines are not to be interrupted except for lipids that may be piggybacked into the TPN line. It is highly recommended that flow rates be maintained by an electronic infusion pump (EIP).

- Check vital signs. Use vital signs measurements as a baseline for future comparison of vital signs.

- Check laboratory results, especially serum electrolyte and blood glucose levels. These values will be used for comparison with future laboratory results.

- Assess nutritional status, weight, energy level, and skin changes.

Diagnoses

- *Risk for Infection,* related to TPN therapy, concentrated glucose solutions, and invasive lines requiring dressing and tubing changes.

- *Risk for Fluid Volume Deficit,* related to inadequate fluid intake and osmotic diuresis.

- *Fluid Volume Excess,* related to excess fluid infusion or a health condition that is unable to tolerate a high concentration solution administered at an increased rate.

- *Ineffective Breathing Pattern,* related to complications of central venous lines and fluid volume excess.

- *Knowledge Deficit,* related to unfamiliarity with TPN therapy and procedures specific to IV therapy equipment.

Interventions

- Change IV tubing according to agency policy (usually every 24 to 48 hours). To prevent an air embolus when changing the IV tubing, either clamp the central venous line (use plastic or padded clamps only) or have the client perform the Valsalva maneuver while changing tubing. If an air embolus is suspected, immediately place the client in a Trendelenburg position on his or her left side.

- Never use an existing TPN line for blood samples.

- Place prepared solutions not in use in the refrigerator (remove the solution 2 hours before hanging). TPN is usually started at 1000 mL for the first 24 hours and is increased at a rate of 500 to 1000 mL daily until the desired volume is reached. When discontinuing TPN, decrease the daily rate gradually over 12 to 72 hours according to the order.

- Change central venous line dressings according to hospital policy, usually every 24 to 72 hours using strict sterile technique.

- Monitor the central venous line infusion site for signs of infection or thrombus. Complaints of pain, numbness, or tingling in the fingers, neck, or arm on the same side as the catheter may indicate a thrombus formation. Elevated temperature and labored or rapid breathing, pain, redness, swelling, and drainage at the infusion site are indicators of infection and/or phlebitis.

- Check for signs of pulmonary edema such as dyspnea.

- Observe for signs and symptoms of reactions to lipid solutions; e.g., elevated temperature, flushing, sweating, pressure sensation over eyes, nausea or vomiting, headache, chest or back pain, and dyspnea.

Evaluation/Outcome

- Evaluate the effects of total parenteral nutrition on providing adequate or increased nutrition, i.e., weight increase, fluid and electrolyte balance, and osmolality levels within normal range.

- Client remains free of complications, i.e., infection, air embolism, pulmonary embolism, pulmonary edema.

- Maintain a support system.

Fluid, Electrolyte, and Acid-Base Imbalances in Clinical Situations

▌ INTRODUCTION

In the clinical and chronic care settings, health professionals provide care for persons experiencing a variety of problems related to fluid, electrolyte, and acid-base imbalances. This unit addresses five clinical situations. The first two situations focus on developmental issues related to infants and children and to the aging adult. The remaining chapters focus on acute disorders, gastrointestinal surgical interventions, and the chronic diseases congestive heart failure, diabetic ketoacidosis, and chronic obstructive pulmonary disease. To assess clients' needs and to provide the appropriate care needed for persons with selected health problems, the health professional must have a working knowledge and understanding of concepts related to fluid and electrolyte balance. Knowledge of these concepts allows the health professional to assess physiologic changes that occur with fluid, electrolyte, and acid-base imbalances and to plan appropriate interventions to assist clients as they adapt to these changes.

In each of these chapters, the pathophysiology (physiologic changes), etiology, clinical manifestations, clinical management, clinical considerations, and client management (assessment, diagnoses, interventions, and evaluations/outcome) are included. Clinical considerations summarize important facts related to the fluid, electrolyte, and acid-base problems for the specific health disorder. These considerations should be useful to health care providers when providing care for clients.

Fluid Problems in Infants and Children

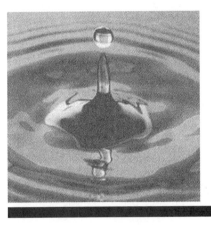

▌ INTRODUCTION

The health professional's understanding of the physiologic differences in infants and children that have implications for fluid and electrolyte balance is essential to providing optimal health care. Since these physiologic differences vary significantly throughout infancy and childhood, important regulatory factors must be viewed in terms of the maturity of the infant or child when addressing fluid balance problems that can be life-threatening in this vulnerable age group.

▌ PATHOPHYSIOLOGY

Neonates, infants, and young children exhibit major physiologic differences from adults in their total body surface area, immature renal structures and endocrine system, and high rate of metabolism affecting hemostatic control. Each of these factors predisposes them to develop-

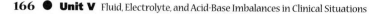

Table 15-1

Comparison of Fluid Volumes to Body Weight in Infants, Children, and Adults

	Embryo	Low Birth Weight Infants	Infants and Children	Adults
Total Weight	97%	80–90%	77% (60% at 1 year)	60%
ECF Volume			50%	20%

mental variations in fluid and electrolyte balance. Water distribution in the newborn or infant is not the same as in an adult. Infants' proportionately higher ECF volume to ICF volume predisposes them to rapid fluid losses, increasing their vulnerability to dehydration. Table 15-1 compares the percent of an individual's fluid volume to body weight over the life span.

Table 15-2 outlines important physiologic differences in infants and children that predispose them to fluid balance problems. The combination of these differences stimulates the metabolic processes of infants and young children to respond to even small changes in fluid volume, resulting in electrolyte imbalances. Untreated imbalances may have major health consequences for this age group. These differences are developmental in nature. As the infant grows and matures, these differences are corrected.

As the child grows, there is muscle growth and cellular growth. More water shifts from the ECF to the ICF compartment. At 1 year, the percentage of the child's total body water is close in amount to the percentage of the adult's (60%) total body water; however, the proportion of ECF and ICF is still different. Generally, serum electrolyte levels in infants and children are similar to adult levels. However, the serum sodium level in newborns fluctuates significantly during the first two days of life.

▶ ETIOLOGY

The etiology of infants' and children's increased risk for fluid balance problems is often complicated by their small size, the immaturity level of

Table 15-2

Physiological Differences in Infants that Predispose Them to Fluid Imbalances

Developmental Physiologic Differences	Pathophysiologic Implications
1. Increased body surface area	Excess water loss via skin (the smaller the infant, the greater the loss) Limited ability to retain water
2. Immature kidneys (can take up to 2 years for kidneys to mature)	Increased water loss (limited ability to retain water)
3. Proportionately higher ratio of ECF volume (50%/wt. compared to 20% in adults)	Predisposes infant to rapid losses of fluid, resulting in dehydration
4. Higher metabolic rate	Predisposes infant to more rapid use of water
5. Immature endocrine system	Limits rapid response of appropriate regulatory system
6. Increased pH in newborns (lasts a few days to a few weeks or may persist in low birth weight infants)	Indicative of metabolic acidosis

various body regulatory systems, their overall health status, and the extent of their fluid reserve. The most common fluid problem in infants and children is a fluid volume deficit. Table 15-3 describes some common fluid and electrolyte problems and etiological factors experienced by infants and children.

▶ CLINICAL MANIFESTATIONS

Signs and symptoms of fluid imbalance vary with the infant's or child's level of maturity, state of hydration, and the source of the problem.

Fluid intoxication from overhydration occurs when excessive fluid ingestion results in low serum sodium levels and central nervous system irritation. Infants are especially vulnerable since their thirst mechanism and kidneys are not well-developed. The typical signs, symptoms, and laboratory findings in overhydration are shown in the accompanying box at the bottom of page 169.

Table 15-3

Common Fluid and Electrolyte Balance Problems with Related Etiological Factors

Problems	Etiological Factors
1. Hyponatremia (Na depletion)	Increased metabolic rate Immature kidneys Fever Malnutrition/diet Excessive insensible water loss Disease states (renal, diabetes, burns) Excessive intake of electrolyte-free solutions Low sodium intake Vomiting/diarrhea Overhydration
2. Hypernatremia (Na excess)	High salt intake (internal or IV) Disease states (renal, diabetes insipidus, hypoglycemia) High insensible water loss Fever
3. Hypokalemia (K depletion)	Malnutrition Malabsorption Cellular breakdown from injury Disease states (renal, GI disorders, diabetes, dehydration acidosis) Burns IV replacement therapy without potassium supplements Selected medications (steroids)
4. Hyperkalemia (K excess)	Disease states (renal, adrenal insufficiency, metabolic acidosis, burns, severe dehydration)
5. Hypocalcemia (Ca depletion)	Inadequate diet Vitamin D deficiency Disease states (renal insufficiency, hypoparathyroidism, alkalosis, GI disorders) Selected medications (diuretics)
6. Hypercalcemia (Ca excess)	Prolonged immobilization Excessive IV or oral administration Disease states (associated with bone catabolism, hypoproteinemia, hypervitaminosis D, hyperparathyroidism, hyperthyroidism, kidney disease)

continues on the following page

Table 15-3

(Continued)

Problems	Etiological Factors
7. Inappropriate antidiuretic hormone secretion (SIADHS) syndrome	CNS injuries Disease states (renal, head injuries, pneumonia, neplasims) Stress Surgery Selected medications (narcotics, barbiturates)
8. Water (dehydration) depletion	Inadequate fluid intake Disease states (GI, renal, diabetes) Immaturity of body regulatory systems Excessive insensible water loss Radiant warmers/phototherapy Improper diuretics dosage Inadequate replacement therapy
9. Overhydration (water excess)	Intake in excess of output (hypertonic fluid overload) Failure to adequately excrete water due to disease states (kidney, heart pump, malnutrition)

Signs, Symptoms, and Laboratory Findings in Overhydration

Signs and Symptoms

1. Edema (may be difficult to detect)
   Moist rales or crackles in lungs
   Hepatomegaly
   Generalized in nature
2. Weight gain (rapid gain of more than 10% of body weight)
3. CNS disturbances
   Irritability, headache, seizure activity, coma
4. Bulging fontanels in infants
5. Lethargy
6. May have excessive urine output
7. Slow bounding pulse
8. Elevated venous pressure
9. Increased spinal fluid pressure

Laboratory Findings

Low urine specific gravity
Decreased serum electrolytes
Decreased hematocrit
Variable urine volume

Dehydration is the most common type of fluid balance problem in infants and children. It occurs when the total amount of fluid output exceeds the total fluid intake. Dehydration associated with diarrhea is the number one cause of fluid and electrolyte imbalance in infants and children. When vomiting occurs with diarrhea, fluid and electrolyte losses are more severe.

Losses in body weight can be used to determine the degree of body fluid loss. For every 1% of weight loss, 10 mL/kg of body fluid is lost. Dehydration is classified as mild, moderate, or severe based on body loss measurements. Table 15-4 outlines the types, clinical manifestations, and suggested interventions for dehydration. Table 15-5 (see page 174) provides guidelines to assess the degree of dehydration in infants and children.

▶ CLINICAL MANAGEMENT

Regardless of the type of fluid volume problem, immediate treatment of infants and children is needed to prevent hypovolemic shock and serious complications such as central nervous system disturbances. Oral rehydration is the treatment of choice for children with mild to moderate dehydration.

For mild dehydration, parents should be urged to give the child any kind of oral fluid that the child tolerates and to continue feedings as tolerated. Formula can be given to infants. If these approaches are unsuccessful, then oral electrolyte solutions should be given.

Table 15-6 (see page 174) contains a list of oral electrolyte solutions that are used for rehydration and maintenance. Generic brands that are similar to Pedialyte are also available. When purchasing generic brands, however, it is important to select the appropriate solution for the type of rehydration or maintenance therapy needed.

Once rehydration is accomplished, the child should be encouraged to resume a normal diet. Some physicians prescribe diluted or lactose-free formulas for infants while others believe full-strength formula can be given. Feedings for breast-fed infants may be supplemented with an electrolyte solution (usually 100 mL/kg is recommended). Any ongoing losses (through stool or emesis) should also be replaced. For each loss through diarrhea stools, 10 mL/kg of the child's body weight should be replaced with an electrolyte solution.

With the resumption of a normal diet, physicians may prescribe 100 mL/kg of an oral electrolyte solution to supplement the diet. Diets that are low in simple carbohydrates and contain easily digestible foods such as cereal, yogurt, cooked vegetables, and soups can be given to older children. Toddlers may tolerate soft or pureed foods. The BRAT diet (bananas, rice, apples, and toast or tea) is no longer recommended because of its limited nutritional value and high carbohydrate, low electrolyte

Table 15-4

Types of Dehydration: Isonatremic, Hypernatremic, and Hyponatremic

Types of Dehydration	Water and Sodium Loss	Serum Sodium Level	ECF and ICF Loss	Causes	Symptoms	Treatment
Isonatremic dehydration (iso-osmolar or isotonic dehydration)	Proportionately equal loss of water and sodium	130–150 mEq/L	Extracellular fluid volume is markedly decreased (severe hypovolemia). Since sodium and water loss are approximately the same, there is no osmotic pull from ICF to ECF. The plasma volume is significantly reduced and shock occurs from decreased circulating blood volume. ICF volume remains virtually constant.	Diarrhea, vomiting, and malnutrition (decreases in fluid and food intake) are the most common causes.	With severe fluid loss, symptoms are characteristic of hypovolemic shock: rapid pulse rate, rapid respiration; later, a decreasing systolic blood pressure. Other symptoms are weight loss, irritability, lethargy, pale or gray skin color, dry mucous membranes, reduced skin turgor, sunken eyeballs, sunken fontanels, absence of tearing and salivation, and decreased urine output.	Fluid should be restored rapidly to correct hypovolemic shock. Iso-osmolar solutions, i.e., Ringer's lactate and 5% dextrose in 0.2% NaCl or 0.3% NaCl, are some of the choices. Replacement should be calculated over 24 h; if dehydration is severe, half of the amount of solution should be given the first 8 h and the remaining half over the next 16 h.

continues on the following page

171

Table 15-4

(Continued)

Types of Dehydration	Water and Sodium Loss	Serum Sodium Level	ECF and ICF Loss	Causes	Symptoms	Treatment
Hypernatremic dehydration (hyperosmolar or hypertonic dehydration) (second leading type of dehydration in children)	Water loss is greater than sodium loss; sodium excess	↑ 150 mEq/L	ECF and ICF volumes are both decreased. Increased ECF osmolality (solutes) results in a shift of fluid from the ICF to the ECF, causing severe cellular dehydration. ECF depletion may not be as severe as ICF depletion. Loss of hypo-osmolar fluid raises the osmolality of ECF.	Severe diarrhea (water is lost in excess to solutes) and high solute intake with decreased water intake are the two most common causes. Others include fever, poor renal function, rapid breathing, or any combination of these conditions.	Shock is less apparent since ECF loss is not as severe. Symptoms include weight loss, avid thirst, confusion, convulsions, tremors, thickened and firm skin turgor, sunken eyeballs and fontanels, absence of tearing, moderately rapid pulse, moderately rapid respirations, frequently normal blood pressure, normal to decreased urine output, and intracranial hemorrhage.	The goal is to increase the ICF and ECF volumes without causing water intoxication. Giving excessive hypo-osmolar solutions or only 5% dextrose in water dilutes ECF, causing water to shift to the ICF and water intoxication (ICF volume excess) to occur. A gradual reduction over 48 h of solution is safest. Dextrose 5% with 0.2% NaCl may be ordered, and later, lactated Ringer's solution. With normal urinary flow, potassium can be added to the solution (2–3 mEq/kg).

Table 15-4

(Continued)

Types of Dehydration	Water and Sodium Loss	Serum Sodium Level	ECF and ICF Loss	Causes	Symptoms	Treatment
Hyponatremic dehydration (hypo-osmolar or hypotonic dehydration)	Sodium loss is greater than water loss; excess water	↓ 130 mEq/L	ECF is severely decreased, and ICF is increased. The osmolality of ECF is lower than the osmolality of ICF. Water shifts from the ECF to the ICF (lesser to the greater concentration). The cerebral cells are frequently affected first as the excess water interferes with brain cell activity.	Severe diarrhea (sodium is lost in excess of water), excessive water intake, electrolyte-free fluid infusions (5% dextrose in water), sodium-losing nephropathy, and diuretic therapy.	Thirst, weight loss, lethargy, comatose, poor skin turgor, clammy skin, sunken and soft eyeballs, absence of tearing, shock symptoms (rapid pulse rate, rapid respirations, and low systolic blood pressure), and decreased urine output.	Ringer's lactate or 5% dextrose in 0.45% NaCl (1/2 NSS) can help to correct the serum sodium level (125–135 mEq/L). For serum sodium of 15 mEq/L, normal saline can be used. For serum sodium of 15 mEq/L or less, 3% saline may be indicated. Rapid fluid correction with electrolytes can cause an excessive shift of cellular fluid into the plasma. The result can be overhydration and congestive heart failure.

Table 15-5

Clinical Assessment of Degrees of Dehydration in Infants and Children

% Dehydration (mL/kg)		
Infants	**Children**	**Clinical Assessment**
5% (50 mL/kg)	3% (30 mL/kg)	Heart rate (10–15% above baseline) Slightly dry mucous membranes Concentrated urine Sunken eyeballs Alert, restless
10% (100 mL/kg)	6% (60 mL/kg)	Increased severity of above Systolic blood pressure may be low Respirations may be deep and increased Urine reduced and concentrated Decreased skin turgor Sunken anterior fontanel Restless or lethargic Irritable to touch
15% (150 mL/kg)	9% (90 mL/kg)	Marked severity of preceding signs Decreased systolic blood pressure Delayed capillary refill Very deep rapid breathing Significant decrease in urine output Decreased level of consciousness

Source: Adapted from *The Harriet Lane Handbook: A Manual for Pediatric House Officers* (14th ed., p. 218), St. Louis: Mosby. Additional data from Samson & Ouzts (1996), p. 394.

Table 15-6

Oral Electrolyte Solutions

Product	Na (mEq/L)	K (mEq/L)	Cl (mEq/L)	Base (mEq/L)	Glucose (g/L)
Infalyte	50	25	45	30	30
Naturalyte	45	20	35	48	25
Pedialyte	45	20	35	30	25
Ricelyte	50	25	45	34	30
Rehydralyte	75	20	65	30	25
ORS (WHO)	90	20	80	30	20

Source: Adapted from *Seminars in Pediatric Infectious Disease* (5th ed., p. 231), by J. Snyder, 1994.

composition. Foods to avoid are fried foods, soda, and jello water.

Oral rehydration therapy is replaced with parenteral therapy in infants and children with severe vomiting, gastric distention, and severe dehydration. Emergency treatment of unstable children with severe dehydration is needed to prevent or correct hypovolemic shock. In emergency situations, fluids should be restored rapidly. The amount and rate of fluid replacement to correct the loss and maintain ongoing requirements is based on the following formula.

Fluid Replacement Formula

Percentage of dehydration (fluid loss in mL/kg of body weight) × the child's body weight in kilograms. For the first 8 hours of rehydration, half of the fluid lost plus the required maintenance fluid is replaced. The second half of the required fluid is replaced over the next 16 hours.

For example, the child who weighs 20 kg and has an estimated dehydration level of 10% of his or her total body weight (100 mL/kg) should receive 1000 mL of replacement fluid for the first 8 hours of rehydration, plus 500 mL of maintenance fluid requirements for a total of *1500 mL* of fluid over the first 8 hours. The second half of the deficit and maintenance total is administered more slowly over the next 16 hours of daily rehydration therapy. Continued replacement over the next 48 to 72 hours is based on the calculated maintenance plus the estimated fluid deficit over that period.

The type of intravenous fluid administered is determined by the type of dehydration. With hyponatremia dehydration, fluids are usually replaced and maintained with $D_5W/.05$ NSS. $D_5W/.2\%$ or .3% NSS may be used for rehydration therapy when isonatremic dehydration is suspected. If serum sodium is below 115 mEq/L, a 3% saline solution is indicated.

The severity of hypernatremic dehydration is often difficult to assess because the fluid shifts between the intracellular and extracellular spaces, preserving the circulating volume. Therefore, the potential of giving too much fluid is present. (Refer to Table 15-5 for fluid guidelines when addressing specific levels of dehydration.)

The goal for correcting hypernatremic dehydration is to prevent water intoxication. When correcting hypernatremic dehydration, calcium replacement followed with potassium replacement is indicated when the normal kidney function returns to normal. Serum sodium correction in hypernatremia should not occur any more rapidly than 0.5–1.0 mEq/L/h.

To ensure that serum sodium levels do not decrease too rapidly or too slowly, serum sodium levels should be monitored every 2 to 4 hours and the fluid rate should be adjusted accordingly. Too rapid administration of fluid may lead to cerebral edema. When serum sodium levels reach 120–125 mEq/L, fluid restrictions should be initiated. Although severe dehydration is treated with intravenous therapy, once the fluid and electrolyte imbalances have stabilized, oral rehydration therapy should be initiated.

Clinical Considerations: Infants and Children

- Total body fluid volume (ratios of total volume to percent of body weight vary with age and have significant implications for fluid management). Even small changes have implications for electrolyte balance.
- Ratio of extracellular fluid volume to intracellular fluid volume (varies with degree of fluid imbalance). Note significant differences among infants, children, and adults.
- pH levels (acidosis) differences have specific implications for varying treatment based on the age and maturity of newborns and low birth weight infants.
- Immature development of regulatory mechanisms for control of fluid and electrolyte balance in infants and children (thirst regulation, kidneys, hormones) increases the potential for shock when treating dehydration in infants and children.
- Hydrogen ion concentrations quickly affect pH levels and may be manifested as a central nervous system disorder.

❘ CLIENT MANAGEMENT
Assessment

- Complete a health history of the current problem.

- Complete a head-to-toe assessment of the infant or child to compare your findings with those of the health history and note symptoms of fluid overload or deficit. Refer to table 15-7 for a complete head-to-toe assessment outline.

- Identify potential health problems related to factors associated with fluid and electrolyte balance, such as changes in weight, eating/drinking patterns, urine output, insensible perspiration, respiratory rate, vomiting, diarrhea, irritability, listlessness, skin (turgor,

Table 15-7

Head-to-Toe Assessment of Fluid and Electrolyte Imbalance in Infants and Children

Observation	Assessment	Rationale
Behavior and Appearance	Irritable/restless Anorexia Purposeless movement Unusual cry Lethargic Lethargy with hyperirritability on stimulation Unresponsive (comatose)	Early symptoms of fluid volume deficit are irritability, purposeless movements, and an unusual or high-pitched cry in infants. Young children may experience thirst with restlessness. As dehydration continues, lethargy and unconsciousness may occur.
Skin	Color _____ Temperature _____ Feel _____ Turgor _____	Skin color may be pale (mild), gray (moderate), or mottled (severe) depending on the degree of dehydration. Temperature is usually cold except with hypertonic dehydration where the temperature may be hot or cold. Skin feels dry with isotonic dehydration; clammy with hypotonic dehydration; and thickened and doughy with hypertonic dehydration. Turgor is measured by pinching the skin on the abdomen, chest wall, or medial aspect of the thigh and assessing the rate of skin retraction (elasticity). As dehydration progresses, elasticity decreases from fair to very poor. With hypertonic dehydration, turgor may remain fair. Skin turgor of obese infants or children may appear normal even with a deficit. Undernourishment can cause poor tissue turgor with fluid balance.
Mucous Membranes	Dryness in oral cavity (cheeks and gums) _____ Dry tongue with longitudinal wrinkles _____	The mucous membranes and tongue are dry with a fluid deficit. Sodium deficit causes the tongue to appear sticky, rough, and red. A dry tongue may also indicate mouth breathing. Some medications and vitamin deficiencies cause dryness of mucous membranes. Dryness in the oral cavity membranes (cheeks and gums) is a better indicator of fluid loss.
Eyes	Sunken _____ Tears _____ Soft eyeballs _____	Sunken eyes and dark skin around them may indicate a severe fluid volume deficit. Tears are absent with moderate to severe dehydration. (Tearing is not present until approximately 4 months of age.) Soft eyeballs may indicate isonatremic or hyponatremic dehydration.

continues on the following page

Table 15-7

(Continued)

Observation	Assessment	Rationale
Fontanel	Sunken _____ Bulging _____	Depression of the anterior fontanel is often an indicator of fluid volume deficit. A fluid excess results in bulging fontanel.
Vital Signs Temperature	Admission Temperature _____ Time _____ (1) _____ Time _____ (2) _____	Body temperature can be subnormal or elevated. Fever increases insensible water loss. The child's extremities may feel cold because of hypovolemia (fluid volume deficit), which decreases peripheral circulation. A subnormal temperature may be due to reduced energy output.
Pulse	Admission pulse _____ Pulse rate Time _____ (1) _____ Time _____ (2) _____ Pattern _____	A weak and rapid pulse rate (over 160 for infant and over 120 for child) may indicate a fluid volume deficit (hypovolemia) and the possibility of shock. A full, bounding, not easily obliterated pulse may indicate a fluid volume excess. An irregular pulse can be due to hypokalemia. A weak, irregular, rapid pulse may indicate hypokalemia, while a weak, slow pulse may indicate hypernatremia.
Respiration	Admission rate _____ Respiration Time _____ (1) _____ Time _____ (2) _____ Pattern _____	Note the rate depth and pattern of the infant's breathing. Dyspnea and moist rales usually indicate fluid volume excess. Rapid breathing increases insensible fluid loss from the lungs. Rapid, deep, vigorous breathing (Kussmaul breathing) frequently indicates metabolic acidosis. Acidosis can be due to poor hydrogen excretion by the kidneys, diarrhea, salicylate poisoning, or diabetes mellitus. Shallow, irregular breathing can be due to respiratory alkalosis.
Blood Pressure	Admission BP _____ Blood pressure Time _____ (1) _____ Time _____ (2) _____	Elasticity of young blood vessels may keep blood pressure stable even when a fluid volume deficit is present. Increased blood pressure may indicate fluid volume excess. Decreased blood pressure may indicate severe fluid volume deficit, extracellular shift from the plasma to the interstitial space, or sodium deficit.

continues on the following page

Table 15-7

(Continued)

Observation	Assessment	Rationale
Neurological Signs	Abdominal distention _____ Diminished reflexes (hypotonia) _____ Weakness/paralysis _____ Tetany tremors (hypertonia) _____ Twitching, cramps _____ Sensorium Confusion _____ Comatose _____ Other _____	Abdominal distention and weakness may indicate a potassium deficit. Tetany symptoms can indicate a calcium and/or magnesium deficit. Serum calcium deficits occur easily in children, since their bones do not readily replace calcium to the blood. Confusion can be due to a potassium deficit and/or fluid volume deficit.
Neurovascular Signs	Capillary filling time _____	A measure of systemic perfusion. Moderate to severe dehydration is often accompanied by delayed capillary filling time of >2–3 seconds.
Weight	Pre-illness weight _____ Current weight _____	Weight loss can indicate the degree of dehydration (fluid loss): Mild—2–5% in infants and young children Moderate—5–10% in infants and young children; 3–6% in older children Severe—10–15% in infants and young children; 6–9% in older children Fluid loss can also be estimated by considering that 1 g of weight loss equals 1 mL of fluid loss. Edema and ascites can occur with fluid imbalances. Fluid overloads can result in hepatomegaly (enlarged liver). Weights should be taken on the same scale, at the same time each day, and with the same covering.
Absence of Tearing and Salivation	Absence of tearing _____ Decrease in saliva _____ Absence of saliva _____	Absence of tearing and salivation are indicators of fluid volume deficit. These symptoms occur with moderate dehydration (6–10% body weight loss).
Thirst	Thirst Mild _____ Avid _____	Thirst is an indicator of dehydration (fluid loss). Thirst may be difficult to determine when vomiting is present. If vomiting is present, offer flat carbonated fluid (Coca-Cola or ginger ale). Avid thirst may indicate serum hyperosmolality and cellular dehydration.

continues on the following page

Table 15-7

(Continued)

Observation	Assessment	Rationale
Urine	Number of voidings in 8 h _____ Amt mL/8 h _____ Amt mL/h _____ Urine color _____ Specific gravity _____ Urine pH _____	Accurate measurements of intake and output from all sources is essential. Normal output ranges are: Infants: 2–3 mL/kg/h Young children: 2 mL/kg/h Older children: 1–2 mL/kg/h By subtracting the weight of a saturated urine diaper from a dry diaper, output in infants and toddlers can be determined (1 g wet diaper = 1 mL urine). Because of evaporative losses, diapers must be weighed within 30 min of the void to be accurate. Specific gravity can be obtained by refractometer or dipstick. Accurate assessment can be made within 2 h of the void. Oliguria (decrease in urine output) with very concentrated urine (dark yellow color) and increased specific gravity (>1.020 for infants and 1.030 for children) can indicate a moderate to severe fluid volume deficit, plasma to interstitial fluid shift, sodium deficit or severe sodium excess, potassium excess, or renal insufficiency. An elevated specific gravity is also indicative of glycosuria and proteinuria. With severe fluid deficit the infant may not void for 16–24 h and not show evidence of abdominal distention. Polyuria (increased urine output) with low specific gravity (<1.010) can indicate fluid excess, renal disease, a sodium deficit, or extracellular shift from interstitial fluid to plasma or decreased antidiuretic hormone (ADH). An acidic pH may indicate metabolic or respiratory acidosis, alkalosis with severe potassium deficit, or a fluid deficit. Alkaline urine may result from metabolic or respiratory alkalosis, hyperaldosteronism, acidosis with chronic kidney infection and tubular dysfunction, or diuretic therapy.
Stools	Number _____ Consistency _____ Color _____ Amount _____	The consistency, color, and amount of each stool should be noted. If the stool is liquid, it should be measured. Frequent liquid stools can lead to fluid volume deficit, potassium and sodium deficit, and bicarbonate deficit (acidosis).

continues on the following page

Table 15-7

(Continued)

Observation	Assessment	Rationale
Vomitus	Number _____ Consistency _____ Color _____ Amount _____	Vomitus needs to be described according to consistency, color, and amount. Frequent vomiting of large quantity leads to fluid loss, potassium and sodium loss, as well as hydrogen and chloride loss (alkalosis).

Other Fluid Loss	GI suction
	  Amount _____
	Drainage tube
	  Amount _____
	Fistula
	  Color _____
	  Amount _____
	Other
	  Amount _____
		Fluid loss from all sources should be measured. Fluid loss from GI suctioning, drainage tubes, and fistula can contribute to severe fluid and electrolyte imbalance.

Blood Chemistry and Hematology	Electrolytes
	Time _____ Time _____
	K _____ _____
	Na _____ _____
	Cl _____ _____
	Ca _____ _____
	Mg _____ _____
	BUN _____ _____
	Creatinine
	  _____ _____
	Hgb _____ _____
	Hct _____ _____
		One set of blood chemistry is not sufficient for assessment. Electrolytes should be frequently monitored when they are not in normal range.
		Norms are:
		K:
		  Newborn 3.0–6.0 mEq/L
		  Infant & older 3.5–5.0 mEq/L
		Na:
		  Newborn 136–146 mEq/L
		  Infant 139–146 mEq/L
		  Child 135–148 mEq/L
		Cl:
		  Newborn 97–110 mEq/L
		  Child 98–111 mEq/L
		Ca:
		  Newborn 7–12 mg/dL
		  Child 8–10.8 mg/dL
		Mg:
		  All ages 1.3–2.0 mEq/L
		BUN:
		  Newborn 4–18 mg/dL
		  Child 5–18 mg/dL
		Creatinine:
		  Newborn 0.3–1.0 mg/dL
		  Infant 0.2–0.4 mg/dL
		  Child 0.3–0.7 mg/dL
		Hgb:
		  Newborn 14.5–22.5 g/dL
		  Infant 9–14 g/dL
		  Child 11.5–15.5 g/dL

continues on the following page

Table 15-7

(Continued)

Observation	Assessment	Rationale
		Hct: Newborn 44–72% Infant 28–42% Child 35–45% An elevated BUN can indicate fluid volume deficit or kidney insufficiency. Elevated creatinine frequently indicates kidney damage. Elevated hemoglobin and hematocrit may indicate hemoconcentration caused by fluid volume deficit. If anemia is present, the hemoglobin and hematocrit may appear falsely normal.
	Blood gases pH _____ PaCO$_2$ _____ PaO$_2$ _____ HCO$_3$ _____ BE _____	After the first day of life, normal range for pH is 7.35–7.45. A pH of 7.35 or less indicates acidosis. A pH of 7.45 or higher indicates alkalosis. Newborns and infants have PaCO$_2$ levels that range between 27 and 41 mm Hg. After infancy, PaCO$_2$ levels range from 35 to 48 mm Hg in males and from 32 to 45 mm Hg in females. Lower values indicate respiratory alkalosis or compensation (overbreathing, hyperventilating). Higher values mean respiratory acidosis. Normal range for HCO$_3$ in all ages is 21–28 mEq/L. BE (base excess) varies with age. Normal BE ranges are: Newborn (−10)–(−2) mEq/L Infant (−7)–(−1) mEq/L Child (−4)–(+2) mEq/L HCO$_3$ below 21 and BE less than the normal value for age indicates metabolic alkalosis. HCO$_3$ above 28 and BE higher than the normal value for age indicates metabolic acidosis.

color, temperature), membranes, eyes, tears, fontanels, vital signs, neurological signs, neurovascular measurements, and stool frequency/consistency.

- Complete lab studies on electrolytes (hemoglobin/hematocrit, urine specific gravity) to determine fluid and electrolyte balance problems.

- Obtain a baseline of vital signs, weight, and so on for comparison with future measurements.

Diagnoses

- *Fluid Volume Deficit,* related to decreased fluid reserve or excessive vomiting and diarrhea.
- *Fluid Volume Excess,* related to inadequate fluid excretion and/or alternative fluid volume regulation.
- *Altered Nutrition, less than body requirements,* related to starvation, diabetic ketoacidosis.
- *Knowledge Deficit (parents),* related to the fluid needs of infants and children.

Interventions

Fluid Volume Deficit

- Monitor lab values (creatinine ratio, electrolyte, hemoglobin, hematocrit, urine specific gravity).
- Closely monitor for changes in general appearance, behaviors, and neurologic activity.
- Monitor weight daily.
- Monitor vital signs in accordance with severity of health problems.
- Integrate observations to determine the type (iso-osmolar, hypo-osmolar, hyperosmolar) and degree (mild, moderate, severe) of dehydration.
- Monitor effects of fluid replacement on behavior and laboratory findings.
- Monitor balance in intake and output measures.

Fluid Volume Excess

- Attempt to identify the source of the fluid overload.
- Closely monitor intake and output for imbalance.
- Monitor laboratory values (electrolytes, hemoglobin, hematocrit, urine specific gravity, and creatinine ratio), and report even small changes.
- Monitor vital signs in accordance with severity of the imbalance.
- Monitor weight daily.

- Observe closely for CNS signs and symptoms that may result in seizures or coma.
- Monitor extremities, face, perineum, and torso for signs of edema.
- Provide a quiet, controlled environment.
- Record and report even small changes in findings.

Evaluation/Outcome

- Evaluate that the cause of the fluid volume problem has been eliminated or controlled (disease state identified, vomiting and/or diarrhea controlled, hemorrhage, and so on) and the electrolyte imbalance and/or fluid intake has been adjusted appropriately.
- Evaluate the effectiveness of interventions through selected electrolyte studies (Na, Cl, K, Ca) to verify that they have returned to normal range.
- Document daily weight (in kilograms for infants and young children) for return to stable baseline weight (consult parents if necessary).
- Evaluate general appearance for improvement in signs and symptoms of fluid imbalance (lethargy, hyperirritability, sunken or bulging fontanels in infants, edema, weak/shrill cry, seizures, and so on).
- Monitor for fluid balance through intake and output measures. Document parental understanding of teaching related to the signs and symptoms of dehydration in children.
- Evaluate hydration status (return of moist, pink mucous membranes, good skin turgor, and so on) of infant or child.
- Monitor weight frequently (small gains or losses are significant in infants and children).

Aging Adults with Fluid and Electrolyte Imbalances

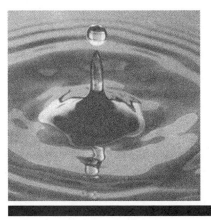

▶ INTRODUCTION

The health professional's understanding of the structural and functional changes in aging adults that have implications for fluid and electrolyte balance is essential to providing optimal health care for this rapidly growing sector of the population. Since the structural and functional changes in the aging adult are often complicated by chronic health problems, the aged are often vulnerable to life-threatening complications. When fluid and electrolyte imbalances occur, health interventions must include careful attention to these imbalances.

▶ PATHOPHYSIOLOGY

Structural and functional changes that occur as a result of the aging process are usually measured in terms of the body's ability to adapt. Additional risk factors such as chronic diseases increase the debilitating

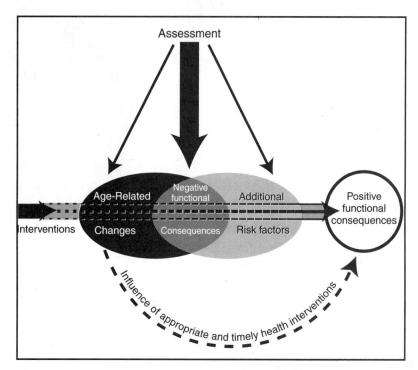

Figure 16-1 Functional Consequences Model of Gerontological Nursing

effects of normal functional changes in all of the body's systems and further inhibit the aging adult's ability to maintain fluid and electrolyte balance. Assessments provide information about age-related changes and factors that may place older adults at risk for fluid and electrolyte imbalances. Miller (1990) proposed the Functional Consequences Model of Gerontological Nursing (Figure 16-1) to show how age-related changes and risk factors such as stress and disease may combine to cause negative functional consequences. Appropriate interventions are needed to foster positive functional consequences and decrease the debilitating effects of these risk factors.

Table 16-1 lists (1) age-related structural and functional changes in five major body systems; (2) health risk factors for fluid and electrolyte imbalance; (3) functional changes resulting from age-related changes and potential risk factors; and (4) interventions to foster positive functional outcomes. Because of these changes, the aged person adapts more slowly, has more difficulty maintaining homeostasis, and has an increased risk for developing a fluid and electrolyte imbalance. Risk factors are complicated by diminished structural and functional efficiency of the aging pulmonary, renal, cardiac, gastrointestinal, and integumentary systems.

Table 16-1

Major Structural Changes, Risk Factors, and Functional Outcomes in Aging Adults

Body System	Structural Changes	Risk Factors	Functional Outcomes	Nursing Interventions
Pulmonary function decreased	Loss of elasticity of parenchymal lung tissue with 20% decrease in weight Increased rigidity of chest wall Fewer alveoli Decreased strength of expiratory muscles	Chronic diseases Emphysema Asthma Chronic bronchitis Bronchiectasis Injuries, smoking Longer sleeping hours Exposure to air pollutants Occupational exposure to toxic substances Infection Decreased immune system response	Defective alveolar ventilation Accumulation of bronchial secretions Increased CO_2 retention Increased difficulty in regulating pH Decreased tolerance for exercise Decreased vital capacity response Increased residual volume	Increase breathing capacity to enhance the elimination of CO_2 by: 1. Breathing exercises with prolonged expiration 2. Coughing after a few deep breaths 3. Frequent position changes 4. Chest clapping 5. Intermittent positive pressure breathing (IPPB)
Renal function decreased	Arteriosclerotic changes in large renal vessels Decrease in number of functioning nephrons (begins by age 40) 30–50% less by age 70 Decrease in size and weight of the kidneys Increased interstitial tissue Decrease in number glomeruli Thickening of glomeruli and tubular membranes Increased potential for development of diverticuli	Medications (e.g., diuretics) Genitourinary diseases (e.g., infections, obstructions)	Reduced glomerular filtration Decreased renal blood flow Impaired ability to excrete water and solutes causing: 1. A decrease in H^+ excretion; thus, metabolic acidosis can occur 2. Reduced ability to concentrate urine 3. Increased accumulation of waste products in body 4. Decreased ability to excrete drugs Decline in urine creatinine clearance Overall decrease in adaptive capacity of the kidneys to stress	Assess adaptive capacity and maintain optimal renal function by: 1. Checking fluid intake and output balance 2. Encouraging fluid intake as appropriate 3. Checking acid-base balance according to serum CO_2 or HCO_3 4. Testing specific gravity to determine kidneys' ability to concentrate urine 5. Noting drugs that may be toxic to renal function 6. Observing for side effects from drug accumulation 7. Observing for desired effects of drugs

continues on the following page

Table 16-1

(Continued)

Body System	Structural Changes	Risk Factors	Functional Outcomes	Nursing Interventions
Circulation and cardiac function decreased	Increased rigidity and decreased elasticity of arterial walls (arteriosclerosis) Decreased elasticity of blood vessels Thickening of cardiac vessels and valves Decrease in number of conductive cells	Obesity Smoking Dietary habits that contribute to risk factors: 　Hyperlipidemia, excess salt and calories Inactivity Low potassium intake Diuretic therapy Excessive alcohol consumption Stress Air pollution Hormone changes	Potential increase in blood pressure Stasis of blood causing back pressure on capillaries, which in turn causes fluid to move into tissue areas causing edema Decreased cardiac output and decreased blood flow Decreased cardiac reserve (capacity of heart to respond to increased burden) slows the adaptive functions as evidenced by: 1. Heart rate same as young adults except under stress takes longer to return to normal 2. Increased incidence of edema and congestive heart failure Diminished strength of cardiac contractions Decreased cardiac output and stroke volume Decreased compensatory responses to blood pressure changes	Assess adaptive capacity of heart and maintain circulation and cardiac function by: 1. Checking blood pressure for elevations resulting from arteriosclerotic changes 2. Determining blood flow by checking peripheral pulses 3. Checking lungs and dependent extremities for edema from increased capillary pressure 4. Checking pulse rates (apical and radial) and character to determine heart contraction, cardiac output, and pulse deficit 5. Noting changes in heart rate following activity 6. Assessing chest sounds for moist rales

Gastrointestinal function decreased	Atrophy of gastric mucosa Muscular atrophy and loss of supportive structures in small intestines	Alcohol or medications Psychosocial factors (e.g., isolation, depression) Factors that interfere with ability to obtain, prepare, consume, or enjoy food and fluids (e.g., immobility, mental impairment) Extraintestinal disorders (diabetes, vascular disorders, and neurologic changes)	Decrease in gastric secretions, especially HCl Metabolic alkalosis related to decreased HCl Atrophic gastritis due to decreased HCl Weakened intestinal wall causing diverticuli Decreased motility (peristalsis) of gastrointestinal tract (may cause constipation) Decreased calcium absorption Decreased solubility and absorption of some drugs	Assess for adaptive changes and maintain gastrointestinal function by: 1. Discussing client preferences for foods 2. Suggesting dietary alterations according to physiologic changes, individual preferences, and nutritional needs; may need increased calcium and vitamin D 3. Encouraging fluid intake 4. Checking frequency, consistency, and stool color in bowel elimination 5. Assessing bowel sounds and level of peristalsis
Liver function and endocrine gland function decreased	Liver cells decrease in size and character Hormonal cells decrease in size and character, and outputs dwindle	Liver or endocrine diseases Medications (e.g., steroids, cardiac medications, antibiotics) Alcohol consumption	Liver: 1. Decreased hepatic capacity to detoxify drugs 2. Decreased synthesis of cholesterol and enzyme activity Hormonal: 1. Decreased overall metabolic capacity 2. Decreased endocrine gland function to react to adverse drug action	Assess adaptive liver and endocrine gland functioning by: 1. Noting drugs client is taking that may be toxic to liver 2. Observing for toxic effects of drug buildup 3. Observing for desired effects of drugs 4. Assessing alcohol consumption and teaching accordingly 5. Assessing for jaundice

continues on the following page

Table 16-1

(Continued)

Body System	Structural Changes	Risk Factors	Functional Outcomes	Nursing Interventions
Skin function decreased	Epidermis—thinner Dermis—thinning and loss of elasticity and strength Blood flow—decreased Sebaceous glands—decreased production Sweat glands—decreased production Decrease in number of nerve endings	Exposure to ultraviolet rays (sunlight) Adverse medication effects Personal hygiene habits (e.g., too frequent bathing) Immobility Friction Chemical Mechanical injury Temperature—too high or low Pressure Gene influence	Drier, coarser skin Increased threshold level to pain and temperature sensitivity Decreased ability to produce sweat Impaired ability to maintain body temperature	Maintain skin integrity and function by: 1. Maintaining hydration 2. Maintaining optimal skin temperature 3. Maintaining mobility to enhance circulation 4. Turning patient and elevating extremities when necessary to minimize edema and skin breakdown 5. Educating elderly about decreased sensitivity to pain and temperature 6. Providing special mattress or sheepskins for those at risk

▶ ETIOLOGY

Multiple interactive etiological factors increase the aging adult's risk for fluid and electrolyte imbalances. In addition to the many structural and functional changes of the aging process outlined in Table 16-1, the aged adult's ability to adapt to changes in fluid and electrolyte balance is often complicated by chronic disease, stress, depression, and/or medications that interfere with fluid and electrolyte balance. Refer to Table 16-2 for a summary of fluid problems in the aging adult.

▶ CLINICAL MANIFESTATIONS

Signs and symptoms of fluid and electrolyte imbalances in the aged vary with the individual's ability to maintain a fluid reserve, the efficiency of the individual's regulatory systems (heart, lungs, kidney, GI, liver, endocrine, and skin), and any complicating disease factors or weight problems. Since structural changes and related aging risk factors influence the manifestation of clinical symptoms as functional clinical changes, it is important to view health problems in terms of each system affected, structural changes, and related risk factors when attempting to diagnose and treat presenting symptoms. Table 16-3 outlines typical presenting symptoms of an 89-year-old, frail elder, experiencing a fluid volume excess. Table 16-4 (see page 197) outlines some typical presenting symptoms for a 67-year-old, semi-independent male, experiencing a fluid volume deficit. Note the relationship of structural aging changes, risk factors, and functional outcomes in each example.

Table 16-2

Body Fluid Problems in the Aging Adult

Problems	Etiology	Interventions
Fluid Volume Deficit: Dehydration	1. Insufficient water intake 2. Increased urinary output 3. Decreased thirst mechanism 4. Diminished response to ADH (antidiuretic hormone) 5. Reduced ability to concentrate urine	1. Measure fluid intake and output to assess fluid balance 2. Encourage adequate oral fluid intake 3. Assess osmolality of IV fluid intake 4. Assess for clinical signs and symptoms of hypovolemia (dehydration) 5. Monitor other types of fluid therapy, e.g., IV clysis and tube feeding. Adjust rate of IV fluid according to age and physiologic state

continues on the following page

Table 16-2

(Continued)

Problems	Etiology	Interventions
Fluid Volume Excess Edema	1. Slightly elevated ECF 2. Overhydration from IV therapy 3. Increased capillary pressure 4. Cardiac insufficiency	1. Measure fluid intake and output to assess fluid balance 2. Adjust IV flow rate to prevent overhydration 3. Assess for peripheral edema in morning 4. Assess chest sounds for moist rales 5. Observe for signs and symptoms of hypervolemia—overhydration
Water intoxication	1. Hypo-osmolar solutions with copious amounts of drinking water	1. Assess types of IV fluids, e.g., 5% dextrose in water replacement to prevent complications 2. Observe for signs and symptoms of water intoxication 3. Check laboratory results for osmolar effects (Hgb, Hct, electrolytes, BUN)
Alternate Bowel Elimination: Constipation	1. Decrease in water intake 2. Muscular atrophy of small and large intestines with decrease in GI motility 3. Perceptual loss of bowel stimulation	1. Encourage fluid intake 2. Assess bowel sounds for peristalsis 3. Administer mild laxative, and teach dangers of abuse 4. Have patient eat at regular times 5. Offer bedside commode 6. Increase roughage in diet as tolerated 7. Observe color, consistency, and frequency of stools
Alternate Bowel Elimination: Diarrhea	1. Tube feedings with too much carbohydrate 2. Constipation—with small amount of liquid stools 3. Partially digested nutrients 4. Viral or bacterial infection	1. Assess for problem causing diarrhea 2. Administer drug(s), e.g., Lomotil, Kaopectate, to decrease motility of bowel 3. Observe color, frequency, and consistency of stool

Diaphoresis	1. Excessive perspiration
	  a. Fever
	  b. High environmental temperature and/or humidity
		1. Identify cause of problem

Table 16-3

Characteristics of an Aging Client with ECFVE

Body System Affected	Structural Changes	Risk Factors	Functional Changes	Diagnoses	Interventions	Rationale
Cardiac	Arteriosclerosis Increased capillary pressure Decreased effectiveness of cardiac contractions	Recent weight gain of 10 pounds Low protein intake	High blood pressure Edema Decreased cardiac output Increased heart rate	Fluid volume excess: edema, related to decreased cardiac output as evidenced by taut, shiny skin	1. Monitor intake and output, body weight, vital signs, and neck veins for distension 2. Monitor hemoglobin and hematocrit 3. Administer diuretics as ordered by physician 4. If on diuretics, monitor K⁺	Checking for overhydration is important to measure the effectiveness for medical treatment and interventions Hemoglobin and hematocrit concentration are important to assess fluid balance changes A↓ Hgb and Hct levels can indicate fluid overload Diuretics increase fluid loss and decrease edema. Many diuretics cause potassium loss

continues on the following page

Table 16-3

(Continued)

Body System Affected	Structural Changes	Risk Factors	Functional Changes	Diagnoses	Interventions	Rationale
Respiratory	Loss of elasticity of the parenchymal lung tissue Increased rigidity of the chest wall	Immobility Exertion Hypoventilation	CO_2 retention Respiratory acidosis and Reduced breathing capacity	Risk for respiratory insufficiency Impaired gas exchange Ineffective breathing patterns	1. Monitor chest for adventitious sounds 2. Observe for cough, which may indicate pulmonary edema 3. Breathing exercises—prolonged expiration 4. Coughing after a few deep breaths 5. Change position frequently 6. Chest clapping	To assess for fluid overload Cough is an early sign of fluid overload Assists in removing excess CO_2 To enhance gas exchange $(O_2 + CO_2)$ Assists in lung expansion Loosens mucus
Renal	Persistent renal vasoconstriction from arteriosclerotic changes and decreased numbers of functioning nephrons	Medications Genitourinary obstructions	Reduced glomerular filtration rate and ability to excrete water and solute	Fluid volume deficit related to decreased fluid intake	1. Assess intake and output 2. Encourage oral fluids as tolerated 3. Assess acid-base balance 4. Assess urine specific gravity (SG)	To determine amount of excess fluid loss Assists with fluid replacement To observe for metabolic changes Increased urine SG indicates inadequate fluid intake or decreased renal function

| Gastrointestinal | Atrophy of gastric mucosa
Loss of supportive structure of small and large bowel | Immobility
Medications | Decreased mobility of GI tract
Loss of perception of signs for bowel elimination | Risk for constipation related to decreased fluid volume, age-related changes, and immobility | 1. Encourage fluids as tolerated
2. Increase mobility as tolerated
3. Encourage proper diet to ensure elimination
4. Assess bowel sounds
5. Check frequency of bowel elimination and consistency of stools | To assist with proper bowel elimination
Physical mobility enhances GI mobility
A balanced diet with fiber enhances bowel elimination
To determine functional status of the GI system
To determine risk of bowel complications |

continues on the following page

Table 16-3
(Continued)

Body System Affected	Structural Changes	Risk Factors	Functional Changes	Diagnoses	Interventions	Rationale
Liver* Integumentary	Loss of elasticity and strength of skin Decreased blood flow, sebaceous and sweat gland production	Edema Immobility	Taut, shiny skin reduces protective function	Impaired skin integrity related to edema and immobility	1. Avoid friction, prolonged pressure, chemical irritation, mechanical injury, excessive temperature variations	To reduce possible skin breakdown due to edema and/or immobility
					2. Encourage mobility to enhance circulation	Good circulation improves skin repair
					3. Raise extremities	To improve circulation and reduce edema
					4. Implement interventions for fluid volume excess and pulmonary congestion (PC) respiratory insufficiency	Fluid balance reduces risks to integumentary system

*Not applicable

Table 16-4

Characteristics of an Aging Client with ECFVD

Body System Affected	Structural Changes	Risk Factors	Functional Changes	Diagnoses	Interventions	Rationale
Cardiac*						
Respiratory*						
Renal	Persistent renal vasoconstriction Decreased number of functioning nephrons	Obstructions Disease Medications	Decreased thirst mechanism Reduced glomerular filtration rate Decreased ability to excrete water and solute	Fluid volume deficit related to decreased desire to drink fluids secondary to high alcohol intake and social isolation, as evidenced by dry lips, furrowed tongue, and decreased skin turgor	1. Observe for decreased skin turgor, decreased urine output 2. Measure intake and output 3. Check specific gravity of urine 4. Observe lab results for increased red blood cell count, hematocrit, and hemoglobin	Decreased skin turgor is a sign of dehydration. Decreased urine output may be due to dehydration or renal dysfunction To determine fluid balance To assess renal function Provide clues to extent of fluid deficit

continues on the following page

Table 16-4

(Continued)

Body System Affected	Structural Changes	Risk Factors	Functional Changes	Diagnoses	Interventions	Rationale
Gastrointestinal	Muscular atrophy and loss of supportive structure of small and large intestine Atrophy of gastric mucosa	Alcohol intake Poor diet Immobility Decreased motivation to drink fluids other than alcohol Social isolation	Decreased GI secretions Decreased motility Constipation	Potential complication: gastrointestinal bleeding Colonic constipation related to inadequate intake of food and fluids and lack of exercise, as evidenced by infrequent bowel movements, small, hard stools	1. Increase fluid intake of water and fluids 2. Assess fluid balance 3. Encourage a balanced diet with increased roughage 4. Assess bowel sounds 5. Observe color and consistency of stools 6. Hemoccult stools	To enhance bowel elimination and soften stools Fluid balance reduces risk for constipation Balanced diet with fiber stimulates bowel elimination To assess for constipation and/or bleeding Observe for GI bleeding to assess GI motility
Liver	Atrophy of liver cells	Heavy alcohol use Aspirin Social isolation		Potential complication: gastrointestinal bleeding	1. Observe for accumulation of fluids in third spaces	Liver damage can cause fluid shift, e.g., ascites
Integumentary*						

*Not applicable

Table 16-5

Clinical Management of Fluid Balance in the Aging Client

- Adjust fluid and electrolyte replacement therapy to match the aged client's reduced functional efficiency and slower response rate (renal, cardiac, pulmonary, GI, integumentary, and regulatory systems).
- Alert client to side effects of diuretics and other medications and his or her increased risk for fluid and electrolyte imbalances (especially sodium and potassium).
- Educate client to the potential for potassium and fluid deficits related to inappropriate use of laxatives and enemas.
- Recognize client's increased risk for fluid and electrolyte complications in acute illness or surgical interventions.
- Encourage client to select appropriate foods and fluids in balanced quantities to meet individual hydration needs.

❯ CLINICAL MANAGEMENT

Effective management of fluid and electrolyte imbalances for the aged client requires the health professional to integrate findings from their structural and functional assessments with health data related to individual risk factors and chronic diseases that may influence the client's ability to adapt. Once this data is put into perspective, fluid balance can be managed by targeting outcomes appropriate to the client's age-related changes and current health problems. Table 16-5 lists actions to be taken in the clinical management of fluid balance in the aging client.

● Clinical Considerations: Aging Adults

1. Inefficiency of body systems (renal, cardiac, pulmonary, GI, integumentary, and regulatory systems) increases with age and chronic health problems, reducing both the effectiveness and speed of bodily responses to stressors.

2. Hypernatremia associated with fluid imbalance is a common problem for the aging adult. It is usually related to poor fluid consumption and can be associated with tube feedings when high protein feedings are used.

3. Potassium-depleting diuretics tend to induce hypokalemia in the aging adult; potassium-sparing diuretics are more likely to produce hyperkalemia.

4. Diuretic-induced fluid deficits are often associated with orthostatic hypotension.

5. Prolonged use of strong laxatives and enema dependency can cause hypokalemia and fluid volume deficits.

6. Standard colon-cleansing procedures can cause fluid and electrolyte complications in the marginally-hydrated aging client.

7. Calcium deficiencies are often associated with osteoporosis. Risks increase with age and postmenopausal osteoporosis.

8. Heat stroke is more common in the aging adult than in other age groups (age-related mortality rates increase after the age of 70).

9. The aging client is at an increased risk for postsurgical complications (cardiac, pneumonia, and fluid and electrolyte imbalance).

▶ CLIENT MANAGEMENT

Assessment

- Complete an extensive health history with careful attention to fluid and electrolyte balance factors (dehydration, fluid overload, edema, mental clarity, and so on).

- Complete a head-to-toe physical assessment with specific attention to structural and functional changes associated with aging.

- Identify risk factors and potential fluid and electrolyte health problems.

- Complete laboratory studies on electrolytes, hemoglobin/hematocrit ratio, creatinine ratio, and urine specific gravity to identify fluid and electrolyte problems.

- Obtain baseline measurements of vital signs and weight for future reference.

Diagnoses

- *Fluid Volume Deficit,* related to severe imbalance between intake and output.

- *Fluid Volume Excess,* related to inadequate fluid excretion associated with poorly functioning regulatory systems (heart, kidneys, lungs).

- *Altered Nutrition, less than body requirements,* related to inadequate diet and increased alcohol consumption.

Interventions

Fluid Volume Deficit

- Monitor lab values (creatinine ratio, electrolyte, hemoglobin, hematocrit, urine specific gravity).
- Closely monitor for changes in general appearance, behaviors, and neurologic activity.
- Monitor weight daily.
- Monitor vital signs in accordance with severity of health problems.
- Integrate observations to determine the type (iso-osmolar, hypo-osmolar, hyperosmolar) and degree (mild, moderate, severe) of dehydration.
- Monitor effects of fluid replacement on behavior and laboratory findings.
- Monitor balance in intake and output measures.

Fluid Volume Excess

- Attempt to identify the source of the fluid overload.
- Closely monitor intake and output for imbalance.
- Monitor laboratory values (electrolytes, hemoglobin, hematocrit, urine specific gravity, and creatinine ratio), and report even small changes.
- Monitor vital signs in accordance with severity of the imbalance.
- Monitor weight daily.
- Observe closely for CNS signs and symptoms that may result in seizures or coma.
- Monitor extremities, face, perineum, and torso for signs of edema.

Evaluation/Outcome

- Evaluate intake and output for fluid balance.
- Evaluate effectiveness of medications and fluid replacement in treatment.
- Monitor nutritional intake to ensure fluid balance.
- Evaluate body weight and vital signs for return to normal client values.
- Evaluate skin turgor, sensitivity, circulation, temperature, and moisture to reduce effects of risk factors.

- Monitor lab results for Hgb, Hct, Na, Cl, K, and Ca until findings are within normal range.
- Monitor reduction of signs and symptoms related to fluid imbalance.
- Maintain a support system.

Acute Disorders: Trauma and Shock

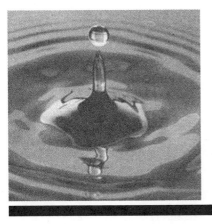

▶ INTRODUCTION

Numerous physiologic changes in fluid and electrolyte imbalances occur as a result of traumatic injuries and shock. Swift and accurate assessment and interventions are necessary to protect the life of the injured client. This chapter is divided into two sections related to fluid, electrolyte, and acid-base changes: trauma and shock.

▶ TRAUMA

Fluid, electrolyte, and acid-base changes occur rapidly in the acutely traumatized client. Quick assessment and action are needed for the best chance of survival. Trauma deaths can occur almost immediately at the time of the trauma, hours later, or days later primarily due to acute respiratory distress syndrome (ARDS), sepsis, or multiple organ failure. Following a traumatic injury, the injured sites are assessed, fluid replacements are prescribed, and medical and/or surgical interventions are performed.

Pathophysiology

Following a severe traumatic injury, there is cellular breakdown (catabolism) due to cell damage and hypoxia. In trauma, sodium shifts into cells and potassium shifts out of cells; fluid shifts from the intravascular (vessels) to the interstitial spaces and cells. These shifts can result in severe fluid and electrolyte imbalances. Kidney activity is altered during and after a severe traumatic injury. Decreased circulatory flow can decrease renal arterial flow and renal perfusion, thus diminishing renal function. With cellular breakdown and hypoxia, nonvolatile acids such as lactic acid increase in the vascular fluid, causing metabolic acidosis. Also, with decreased renal function, hydrogen ion retention occurs, thus contributing to the acidotic state that generally accompanies trauma and shock. Table 17-1 lists the physiologic changes that occur during trauma.

Etiology

Causes of trauma can result from severe injury due to massive blood loss from major arterial vessels, head injuries to the brain (epidural or subdural hematomas) or brain stem, ruptured spleen, liver lacerations, fractures to large bones, chest injury (hemopneumothorax), and crushed injuries to bones and organs of the body.

Clinical Manifestations

The clinical manifestations that frequently occur in traumatic injuries include changes in vital signs and/or behavioral, cardiac conduction, venous, neuromuscular, and integumentary changes. Laboratory test results are a guide to determine fluid, electrolyte, and acid-base changes that are occurring.

The pulse rate may be fast, irregular, or full-bounding. The blood pressure decreases according to the blood volume and fluid deficit. With severe fluid loss, the pulse pressure is narrowed. Tachypnea, dyspnea, or deep and rapid breathing may be present.

To overcome the hypovolemic state caused by blood and fluid loss and fluid shift to the injured site and cells, the syndrome of inappropriate antidiuretic hormone (SIADH) occurs. This is a compensatory mechanism to maintain the vascular fluid. The water reabsorption can be continuous for several days. Urine output is decreased due to excess production of ADH.

The client may be irritable, restless, and confused because of hypoxia and fluid and electrolyte losses. Integumentary changes may not be noted immediately following severe trauma with fluid losses. However, after several hours or a day, the skin turgor can be affected and

Table 17-1

Physiologic Changes Associated with Trauma

Physiologic Changes	Causative Factors
Potassium, sodium, chloride, bicarbonate	Potassium is lost from cells due to catabolism (cellular breakdown). As potassium leaves, sodium and chloride with water shift into the cells. The sodium pump does not function properly (see Chapter 7).
Fluid changes	Fluids along with sodium shift into cells and to the third space (interstitial space—at the injured site). The increased cellular and third-space fluids cause a vascular fluid deficit (dehydration) and hyponatremia.
	Serum osmolality may be normal or increased due to the fluid deficit and excess solutes other than sodium, such as potassium and urea. Remember, sodium influences the osmolality of plasma. (see Chapter 1).
	The volume and composition of extracellular fluid (ECF) fluctuates depending on the number of cells injured and the body's ability to restore balance. Two to three days following injury, fluid shifts from the third space at the injured site back into the vascular space.
Protein changes	Trauma results in nitrogen loss due to increased protein catabolism, decreased protein anabolism, and/or a protein shift with water to the interstitial space. The colloid osmotic pressure is decreased in the vascular fluid and increased in the interstitial fluid (tissues), which causes fluid volume deficit (vascular) and edema.
Capillary permeability	Increased capillary permeability causes water to flow into and out of the cells and into tissue spaces. This contributes to hypovolemia (fluid volume deficit).
Hormonal influence	ADH and aldosterone help to restore the ECF. A vascular fluid deficit and/or increased serum osmolality stimulates ADH secretion, which causes water reabsorption from the distal tubules of the kidneys. In certain traumatic situations (surgery, trauma, pain), SIADH (syndrome of inappropriate ADH) occurs and causes excess water reabsorption from the kidneys.
	Aldosterone is secreted from the adrenal cortex due to hyponatremia and stress. Aldosterone promotes sodium reabsorption from the renal tubules and is reabsorbed with water. Potassium is excreted.

continues on the following page

Table 17-1

(Continued)

Physiologic Changes	Causative Factors
Kidney influence	Kidney activity is altered during and after a severe traumatic injury. Sodium, chloride, and water shift to the injured site, which causes hypovolemia. Decreased circulatory flow can decrease renal arterial flow, which can cause temporary or permanent kidney damage. Decreased kidney function results in hyperkalemia.
Acid-base changes	With cellular breakdown and hypoxia from decreased perfusion, nonvolatile acids (acid metabolites), e.g., lactic acid, increase in the vascular fluid, causing metabolic acidosis.
	Kidneys conserve or excrete the hydrogen ion to maintain the acid-base balance. Decreased kidney function can cause hydrogen retention and acidosis.
	The lungs try to compensate for the acidotic state by blowing off excess CO_2—hyperventilation. Blowing off CO_2 decreases the formation of carbonic acid.

mucous membranes may become dry. Table 17-2 lists the clinical manifestations related to trauma.

Clinical Management

Accurate clinical assessment is vitally important when planning and implementing care. Table 17-3 is a guide that may be used when assessing the client for fluid, electrolyte, and acid-base imbalances. To understand the significance of the assessment, the rationale helps to identify the type of imbalance present.

After an acute injury in which there is blood and fluid loss, intravenous therapy is initiated. Balanced electrolyte solutions (BES) such as normal saline solution (0.9% NaCl) and lactated Ringer's solution are usually started immediately. Oral fluids should not be given until the extent of the injury and the need for surgery is determined. Five percent dextrose in water may be used if a BES is not available. However, if D_5W is used continuously, it dilutes the body's electrolytes and can cause water intoxication; therefore, D_5W is not the choice fluid replacement solution in trauma and shock states.

Table 17-2

Clinical Manifestations Related to Trauma

Clinical Manifestations	Signs and Symptoms
Vital Signs	Increased pulse rate (tachycardia), common with present cardiac condition
Pulse	Irregular pulse rate, full-bounding pulse
Blood pressure	Blood pressure decreases when severe fluid loss occurs Pulse pressure narrows
Respiration	Increased breathing (tachypnea) Dyspnea Deep, vigorous breathing (Kussmaul breathing)
Temperature	Hypothermia commonly associated with shock
Behavioral changes	Irritability, restlessness, and confusion
Cardiac conduction changes	ECG: T wave changes (inverted or peaked), ST segment changes, and cardiac dysrythmias (result of coronary ischemia or potassium imbalance)
Venous changes	Neck and hand vein engorgement No vein engorgement with fluid loss
Renal changes	Hourly urine output decreases
Neuromuscular changes	Muscular weakness
Integumentary changes	Poor skin turgor Dry mucous membrane Edema Diaphoresis Draining wound, exudate
Laboratory Findings Electrolytes ↓ or ↑	Serum potassium, sodium, magnesium, chloride may be decreased or increased
Serum CO_2	Decreased CO_2 indicates metabolic acidosis; increased CO_2 indicates metabolic alkalosis or respiratory alkalosis
BUN ↑	Increased BUN indicates fluid loss or decreased renal function
Serum creatinine ↑	Increased serum creatinine indicates decreased renal function
Arterial blood gases: pH, $PaCO_2$, HCO_3	Decreased pH and HCO_3 indicate metabolic acidosis

Table 17-3

Assessment of Fluid, Electrolyte, and Acid-Base Imbalances in the Traumatically Injured Client

Observation	Assessment		Rationale
1. Vital signs: Pulse	Pulse rate Volume Pattern	_____ _____ _____	Changes in vital signs (VS) are indicators of client's physiologic status. Several VS should be taken and the first reading acts as the baseline for comparison. Pulse rate and pattern should be monitored frequently. Pulse rate >120 may indicate hypovolemia and the possibility of shock. Full-bounding pulse can mean hypervolemia and an irregular pulse can mean hypokalemia.
Blood pressure	Admission BP Time Time	_____ _____	Decrease in BP (systolic and diastolic) may not occur until severe fluid loss has occurred. Several BP readings should be taken, and the first BP reading acts as the baseline for comparison. A drop in systolic pressure can indicate hypovolemia. Pulse pressure (systolic minus diastolic) of <20 can indicate shock.
Respiration	Respiration Pattern	_____ _____	Note changes in rate, depth, and pattern. A rate >32 can indicate hypovolemia. Deep, rapid, vigorous breathing can indicate acidosis as a result of cellular damage and shock. Hyperventilating (fast, shallow breathing) can be due to anxiety or hypoxia. Head injury can produce a wide variety of respiratory patterns.
Temperature	Temperature on admission	_____	Hypothermia is a common finding in shock; an elevated temperature can indicate infection.
2. Behavioral changes	Irritable Apprehensive Restless Confused Delirious Lethargic	_____ _____ _____ _____ _____ _____	Irritability, apprehension, restlessness, and confusion are indicators of hypoxia and later of fluid and electrolyte imbalances (hypovolemia, water intoxication, and potassium imbalance).

continues on the following page

Table 17-3

(Continued)

Observation	Assessment	Rationale

3. Neurologic and neuromuscular signs	Sensorium
	    Confused _____
	    Semiconscious _____
	    Comatose _____
	Muscle weakness _____
	Pupil dilation _____
	Tetany
	    Tremors _____
	    Twitching _____
	    Others _____
		Changes in sensorium can be indicative of fluid imbalance. Tetany can indicate a calcium and magnesium deficit. Hypercalcemia can occur with multiple transfusions of banked blood.

4. Fluid loss	Wound(s) _____
	Urine
	    Number of voidings _____
	    Amount
	        mL/h _____
	        mL/8 h _____
	        mL/24 h _____
	    Color _____
	    Specific gravity _____
	Vomitus
	    Number _____
	    Consistency _____
	    Amount _____
	
	Nasogastric tube
	    Amount—mL/8h _____
	    Amount—mL/24 h _____
	
	Drain(s)
	    Number _____
	    Amount _____
		Note the presence of an open draining wound. Kidneys regulate fluids and electrolytes. Monitoring the urine output hourly is most important. Oliguria can indicate a lack of fluid intake or renal insufficiency due to decreased circulation/circulatory collapse or hypovolemia.
		Frequent vomiting in large quantities leads to fluid, electrolyte (potassium, sodium, chloride), and hydrogen losses. Metabolic alkalosis can occur.
		Gastrointestinal secretions should be measured. Large quantity losses of GI secretions can cause hypovolemia.
		Excess drainage could contribute to fluid loss and should be measured if possible.

5. Skin and mucous membrane	Skin color
	    Pale _____
	    Gray _____
	    Flushed _____
	
	Skin turgor
	    Normal _____
	    Poor _____
	
	Edema—pitting peripheral
	    Feet _____
	    Legs _____
		Pale and/or gray-colored skin can indicate hypovolemia or shock. Flushed skin can be due to hypernatremia, metabolic acidosis, or early septic shock.
		Poor skin turgor can result from hypovolemia/dehydration. This may not occur until 1–3 days after the injury.
		Edema indicates sodium and water retention. Sodium, chloride, and water shift into the cells and to the injury site(s) (interstitial or third space).

continues on the following page

Table 17-3

(Continued)

Observation	Assessment		Rationale
	Dry mucous membranes Sticky secretions	_____ _____	Dry, tenacious (sticky) secretions and dry membranes are indicative of dehydration or fluid loss. This may not occur until 1–3 days after the injury.
	Diaphoresis	_____	Increased insensible fluid loss can result from diaphoresis (excess perspiration). Amount of fluid loss from skin can double.
6. Chest sounds and vein engorgement	Chest rales	_____	The chest should be checked for rales due to overhydration (pulmonary edema) following fluid administration/resuscitation.
	Neck vein engorgement Hand vein engorgement	_____ _____	Neck and hand vein engorgement are indicators of fluid excess. Rales and vein engorgement can occur from excess IV fluids or rapid IV administration.
7. ECG (EKG)	T wave Flat Inverted Peaked	 _____ _____ _____	Flat or inverted T waves indicate cardiac ischemia and/or a potassium deficit. Peaked T waves indicate a potassium excess.
8. Fluid intake	Oral fluid intake Amount mL/8 h mL/24 h Types of IV fluids Crystalloids Colloids Blood	 _____ _____ _____ _____ _____	Oral fluids should not be given until the injury(s) can be assessed. If surgery is indicated, the client should be NPO. Crystalloids, i.e., normal saline, lactated Ringer's, are normally ordered first to restore fluid loss, correct shocklike symptoms, restore or increase urine output, and serve as a lifeline to administer IV drugs.
	Amount mL/8 h mL/24 h mL/h	 _____ _____ _____	Five percent dextrose in water can cause water intoxication (ICF volume excess) and is contraindicated as a resuscitation fluid in shock states.

continues on the following page

Table 17-3

(Continued)

Observation	Assessment		Rationale
9. Previous drug regimen	Diuretics Digitalis Steroids Beta blockers Calcium channel blockers	_____ _____ _____ _____ _____	A drug history should be taken and reported to the physician. Potassium-wasting diuretics taken with a digitalis preparation can cause digitalis toxicity in the presence of hypokalemia. Steroids cause sodium retention and potassium excretion. Long-term steroid use can impair adrenal function in shock states and impair the client's ability to mount a stress response. A steroid bolus or "stress dose" is indicated for steroid-dependent clients. Beta blockers and calcium channel blockers block the effects of the sympathetic nervous system. They may block the compensatory mechanisms for shock.
10. Chemistry, hematology, and arterial blood gas changes	Electrolytes *Serum* K _____ Na _____ Cl _____ Ca _____ Mg _____	*Urine/24 h* K _____ Na _____ Cl _____	Electrolytes should be drawn immediately after a severe injury and used as a baseline for future electrolyte results. (See Chapter 6 for normal values.) Urine electrolytes are compared to serum electrolytes. Normal range for urine electrolytes are: K 25–120 mEq/24 h Na 40–220 mEq/24 h Cl 150–250 mEq/24 h
	Serum CO_2	_____	Serum CO_2 >32 mEq/L indicates metabolic alkalosis and <22 mEq/L indicates metabolic acidosis.
	Osmolality Serum Urine	_____ _____	Serum osmolality >295 mOsm/kg indicates hypovolemia/dehydration and <280 mOsm/kg indicates hypervolemia. Urine osmolality can be 100–1200 mOsm/kg with a normal range of 200–600 mOsm/kg.
	BUN Creatinine	_____ _____	An elevated BUN can indicate fluid volume deficit or kidney insufficiency. Elevated creatinine indicates kidney damage. Normal range: BUN 10–25 mg/dL Creatinine 0.7–1.4 mg/dL

continues on the following page

Table 17-3

(Continued)

Observation	Assessment	Rationale
	Blood glucose _____	Blood sugar increases during stress (up to 180 mg/dL, or higher in diabetics).
	Hbg _____ Hct _____	Elevated hemoglobin and hematocrit can indicate hemoconcentration caused by fluid volume deficit (hypovolemia).
	Arterial blood gases (ABGs)	pH: <7.35 indicates acidosis
	pH _____	and >7.45 indicates alkalosis.
	$PaCO_2$ _____	$PaCO_2$ (respiratory component):
	HCO_3 _____	Norms 35–45 mm Hg
	BE _____	Respiratory acidosis ($\downarrow$ pH, $\uparrow$ $PaCO_2$) may occur due to inadequate gas exchange. A $\uparrow$ pH and $\downarrow$ $PaCO_2$ indicate respiratory alkalosis from hyperventilation.
		HCO_3 (renal component):
		Norms 24–28 mEq/L
		A $\downarrow$ HCO_3 and $\downarrow$ pH mean metabolic acidosis, which is the most common acid-base imbalance following injury from inadequate perfusion and lactic acid production.
		An $\uparrow$ HCO_3 and $\uparrow$ pH mean metabolic alkalosis.
		BE (base excess):
		Norms +2 to −2. Same as bicarbonate.
		A base excess of <−22 (also termed base deficit) is an indication of poor perfusion/inadequate resuscitation.

The client is typed and cross-matched for blood if more than 500 mL of blood is lost. Unless there is a significant loss of blood and fluid, the BES helps to restore fluid loss, increase circulation, and increase the blood pressure.

Excess and/or rapidly administered IV solutions can cause overhydration. Signs and symptoms of overhydration may include constant irritated cough, dyspnea, chest rales, neck vein engorgement, and peripheral edema. A serum osmolality greater than 295 mOsm/kg indicates hypovolemia, and a serum osmolality less than 280 mOsm/kg indicates hypervolemia.

▶ SHOCK

Shock is the state of inadequate tissue perfusion that occurs when the hemostatic circulatory mechanism that regulates circulation fails. Shock can result from trauma because of a large loss of blood and fluid, which results in circulatory failure. Most shock-induced conditions are associated with trauma. A common feature of shock, regardless of the cause, is a low circulating blood volume in relation to vascular capacity. In a shock state, blood loss may not necessarily be from hemorrhaging but may result from "pooling" of blood in body cavities, limiting the amount of blood available to circulate. With shock, the cardiac output is insufficient to provide vital organs and tissues with blood. There are four categories of shock: (1) hypovolemic, which includes hematogenic from hemorrhage; (2) cardiogenic; (3) septic; and (4) neurogenic.

Pathophysiology

The physiologic changes resulting from shock include a decrease in blood pressure; an initial increase in vasoconstriction of the blood vessels, particularly the skin, skeletal muscles, and kidneys but not the cerebral vessels; an increase in heart rate; a decrease in metabolism; and a decrease in renal function. Renal insufficiency can occur when hypotension is prolonged. Systolic blood pressure measurements must be 70 mm Hg and above to maintain kidney function and coronary perfusion.

When the blood pressure is low, the baroreceptors (pressure receptors) in the carotid sinus and aortic arch cause an increase in the systemic vasomotor activity that leads to vasoconstriction and cardiac acceleration to maintain homeostasis. The coronary arteries dilate with a decrease in blood volume. Inadequate oxygenation of cells leads to anaerobic metabolism and the formation of nonvolatile acids such as lactic acid. These changes result in an acid-base imbalance known as metabolic acidosis.

In early shock, fluid is shifted from the interstitial space to the intravascular space in order to compensate for the fluid deficit in the vascular system. As a result of this *early* shift, more fluid in the vascular system increases the venous return to the heart and increases the cardiac output. In *late* shock, fluid is forced from the intravascular space (blood vessels) back into the interstitial spaces (tissues). Table 17-4 describes the physiologic changes resulting from shock.

Table 17-4

Physiologic Changes Resulting from Shock

Physiologic Changes	Rationale
Arterial blood pressure: decreased	Reduced venous return to heart decreases cardiac output and arterial blood pressure (BP). Decrease in BP is sensed by pressoreceptors in carotid sinus and aortic arch, which leads to immediate reflex increase in systemic vasomotor activity. (This center is found in the medulla.) Cardiac acceleration and vasoconstriction occur in order to maintain homeostasis with respect to blood pressure. This may be sufficient for early or impending shock.
Vasoconstriction of blood vessels: increased	Increased sympathetic nervous system activity causes vasoconstriction. Vasoconstriction tends to maintain blood pressure and reduce discrepancy between blood volume and vascular capacity (size). Vasoconstriction is greatest in skin, kidneys, and skeletal muscles and not as significant in cerebral vessels. Coronary arteries actually dilate with a decrease in blood volume. This is a compensatory mechanism to provide sufficient blood to the heart muscle (myocardium) for heart function.
Heart rate: increased	Heart rate is increased to overcome poor cardiac output and to increase circulation. Rapid, thready pulse is often one of the first identifiable signs of shock.
Metabolism: decreased	Fall in plasma hydrostatic pressure reduces urinary filtration. Unopposed plasma colloid osmotic pressure draws interstitial fluid into vascular bed. Blood loss results in loss of serum potassium, phosphate, and bicarbonate. Inadequate oxygenation of cells prevents their normal metabolism and leads to anaerobic metabolism and the formation of nonvolatile acids (acid metabolites), thus lowering serum pH values. With a fall in serum pH and a decrease in HCO_3, metabolic acidosis results. A rise in blood sugar is first seen due to release of epinephrine; later, blood sugar falls due to a decline in liver glycogen.
Kidney function: decreased	Low blood pressure causes inadequate circulation of blood to the kidneys. Renal ischemia is the result of a lack of O_2 to the kidneys. Renal insufficiency follows prolonged hypotension. Systolic blood pressure must be 70 mm Hg and above to maintain kidney function. One of the body's compensatory mechanisms in shock is to shunt blood around the kidneys to maintain intravascular fluid. Deficient blood supply makes tubule cells of kidneys more susceptible to injury. Urine output of less than 25 mL/h may be indicative of shock and/or decrease in renal function.

Etiology

Four types of shock—hypovolemic, cardiogenic, septic (also known as endotoxic or vasogenic), and neurogenic—are named for the clinical cause of the shock conditions. There are four classes of hypovolemic shock based on the amount of blood lost. With Class I there is approximately less than 1 1/2 units of blood loss. Class II may have up to 3 units or 1500 mL of blood loss. Severe shock occurs with Class III (3 to 4 units of blood loss) and Class IV (more than 4 units or 2000 mL of blood loss).

Table 17-5 describes the four types of shock, the clinical causes, and the rationale and physiologic changes that occur with each type. Hemorrhaging from injury or surgery, burns, or GI bleeding can cause hypovolemic shock. Cardiogenic shock may be caused by a myocardial infarction, cardiac failure, or cardiac tamponade. Severe bacterial infection and immunosuppressant therapy contribute to the development of septic shock. Neurogenic shock can result from high spinal anesthesia, severe emotional factors, or trauma from extensive operative procedures.

Clinical Manifestations

Pale, cool skin; apprehension; restlessness; muscle weakness; a fall in blood pressure; tachycardia; tachypnea; and decreased urine output are characteristic signs and symptoms of the four types of shock. In shock, tachycardia is frequently seen before the blood pressure begins to fall. The increased heart rate is an early compensatory mechanism to increase circulation. A low pulse rate (the difference between the systolic and diastolic pressures) of 20 mm Hg or less is indicative of shock. To maintain coronary circulation and renal function, the systolic pressure should be at least 70 mm Hg. Decreased central venous pressure (CVP), pulmonary artery pressure (PAP), and pulmonary capillary wedge pressure (PCWP) are present in all types of shock except septic shock. These pressures may be increased in cardiogenic shock.

Table 17-6 (see page 218) lists the clinical signs and symptoms and rationales related to the four types of shock.

Clinical Management

Immediate action needs to be taken when shock occurs so that it can be reversed. To maintain body fluid volume and particularly the intravascular fluid, fluid replacement must begin immediately for clients who are in shock or impending shock. Improvement of blood volume is needed to maintain tissue perfusion and oxygen delivery. The types of solutions for fluid replacement include crystalloids or balanced electrolyte (salt) solutions, and colloid solutions.

Table 17-5

Types and Clinical Causes of Shock

Type of Shock	Clinical Causes	Rationale and Physiologic Results
Hypovolemic: Hematogenic (from hemorrhage)	Severe vomiting or diarrhea—acute dehydration Burns, intestinal obstruction, fluid shift to third space Hemorrhage that results from internal or external blood loss	Blood, plasma, and fluid loss from decreased circulating blood volume *Physiologic Results* 1. Decreased circulation 2. Decreased venous return 3. Reduced cardiac output 4. Increased afterload 5. Decreased preload 6. Decreased tissue perfusion
Cardiogenic	Myocardial infarction Severe arrhythmias Congestive heart failure Cardiac tamponade Pulmonary embolism Blunt cardiac injury (formerly "cardiac contusion")	Because of these clinical problems, the pumping action of the heart is inadequate to maintain circulation (pump failure of myocardium). *Physiologic Results* 1. Decreased circulation 2. Decreased stroke volume 3. Decreased cardiac output 4. Increased preload 5. Increased afterload 6. Increased venous pressure 7. Decreased venous return 8. Decreased tissue perfusion
Septic: Endotoxic Vasogenic	Severe systemic infections Septic abortion Peritonitis Debilitated conditions Immunosuppressant therapy	Septic shock is characterized by increased capillary permeability that permits blood, plasma, and fluid to pass into surrounding tissue. Often caused by a gram-negative organism. *Physiologic Results* 1. Vasodilatation and peripheral pooling of blood 2. Decreased circulation 3. Decreased preload, early shock and increased preload, late shock 4. Decreased afterload, early shock and increased afterload, late shock. 5. Decreased tissue perfusion

continues on the following page

Table 17-5

(Continued)

Type of Shock	Clinical Causes	Rationale and Physiologic Results
Neurogenic	Mild to moderate neurogenic shock: Emotional stress Acute pain Drugs: narcotics, barbiturates, phenothiazines High spinal anesthesia Acute gastric dilation Severe neurogenic shock: Spinal cord injury Trauma: Extensive operative procedure	Neurogenic shock is caused by loss of vascular tone. *Physiologic Results* 1. Decreased circulation 2. Vasodilatation and peripheral pooling of blood 3. Decreased cardiac output 4. Decreased venous return 5. Decreased tissue perfusion

Crystalloids

Crystalloids expand the volume of the intravascular fluid. The two common types of crystalloids used for fluid replacement are normal saline solution (0.9% sodium chloride) and lactated Ringer's solution. Lactated Ringer's solution contains the electrolytes: sodium, potassium, calcium, and chloride with milliequivalents similar to plasma values. Normal saline solution (NSS) is a popular IV solution used for fluid replacement because it is iso-osmolar with approximately the same milliosmoles as plasma. Excess use of normal saline can increase the serum sodium and chloride levels. The lactate in the lactated Ringer's solution acts as a buffer to increase the pH, thus decreasing the acidotic state. Large quantities of lactated Ringer's solution may cause metabolic alkalosis. If the client has a liver disorder, the lactate is not metabolized into bicarbonate and lactic acid can result. Alternating the crystalloid solutions, such as normal saline solution, and lactated Ringer's solution, usually maintains the body's electrolyte and acid-base balance. Table 17-7 (see page 220) lists the content of the two crystalloids that are used to replace fluid loss during shock.

The crystalloid 5% dextrose and water (D_5W) should NEVER be ordered for *total* fluid replacement during shock. D_5W is an iso-osmolar solution; if it is used continuously in large volumes, the solution in the body

Table 17-6

Clinical Manifestations of Shock

Signs and Symptoms	Types of Shock	Rationale
Skin: pale and/or cold and moist (except when caused by a spinal cord injury)	Hypovolemic Cardiogenic Neurogenic Septic (late)	Pale, cold, and/or moist skin results from increased sympathetic action. Peripheral vasoconstriction occurs and blood is shunted to vital organs. Skin is warm and flushed in early septic shock. Skin is warm and dry in neurogenic shock due to spinal cord injury.
Tachycardia (pulse fast and thready)	Hypovolemic Cardiogenic Septic	Increased pulse rate is frequently one of the early signs, except in neurogenic shock, in which the pulse is often slower than normal. Norepinephrine and epinephrine, released by the adrenal medulla, increase the cardiac rate and myocardial contractibility. Tachycardia, pulse >100, generally occurs before arterial blood pressure falls.
Apprehension, restlessness	Hypovolemic Cardiogenic Septic Neurogenic	Apprehension and restlessness, early signs of shock, result from cerebral hypoxia. As the state of shock progresses, disorientation and confusion occur.
Muscle weakness, fatigue	Hypovolemic Cardiogenic Septic Neurogenic	Muscle weakness and fatigue, which occur early in shock, are the result of inadequate tissue perfusion.
Arterial blood pressure: early, a rise in or normal BP; late, a fall in BP	Hypovolemic Cardiogenic Septic Neurogenic	In early shock, blood pressure rises or is normal as a result of increased heart rate. As shock progresses, blood pressure falls because of a lack of cardiac and peripheral vasoconstriction compensation.
Pulse pressure: narrowed, <20 mm Hg		Narrowing of pulse rate occurs because the systolic BP falls more rapidly than the diastolic BP.

continues on the following page

Table 17-6

(Continued)

Signs and Symptoms	Types of Shock	Rationale
Pressures: CVP, PAP, PCWP—decreased in hypovolemic, septic, neurogenic; increased in cardiogenic	Hypovolemic Cardiogenic Septic Neurogenic	Normal values: 1. Central venous pressure (CVP): 5–12 cm H_2O. With decreased blood volume, CVP <5 cm H_2O. 2. Pulmonary artery pressure (PAP): 20–30 mm Hg systolic, 10–15 mm Hg diastolic. With blood volume depletion or pooling of blood, PAP in hypovolemic <10 mm Hg, septic <10 mm Hg, neurogenic <10 mm Hg. In cardiogenic shock, PAP >30 mm Hg. 3. Pulmonary capillary wedge pressure (PCWP): 4–12 mm Hg. With blood volume depletion or peripheral pooling, the PCWP in hypovolemic, septic, and neurogenic <10 mm Hg and in cardiogenic >20 mm Hg.
Respiration: increased rate and depth (tachypnea)	Hypovolemic Cardiogenic Septic Neurogenic	Increased hydrogen ion concentration in the body stimulates the respiratory centers in the medulla, thus increasing the respiratory rate. Acid metabolites, e.g., lactic acid from anaerobic metabolism increases the rate and depth of respiration. Rapid respiration acts as a compensatory mechanism to decrease metabolic acidosis.
Temperature: subnormal	Hypovolemic Cardiogenic Neurogenic	Body temperature is subnormal in shock because of decreased circulation and decreased cellular function. In septic shock, the temperature is elevated.
Urinary output: decreased	Hypovolemic Cardiogenic Septic Neurogenic	Oliguria (decreased urine output) occurs in shock because of decreased renal blood flow caused by renal vasoconstriction. Blood is shunted to the heart and brain. Urine output should be >25 mL/h.

Table 17-7

Crystalloids

Crystalloids	mEq/L						
	Na	K	Ca	Mg	Cl	Lactate	Gluconate
0.9% NaCl (NSS)	154	—	—	—	154	—	—
Lactated Ringer's	130	4	3	—	109	28	—

becomes hypo-osmolar. This can lead to intracellular fluid volume excess (water intoxication) or cellular swelling.

Intravenous solutions containing calcium, such as lactated Ringer's, should NOT be administered with blood transfusions. The calcium in the solution precipitates when it comes in contact with transfused blood. Normal saline solution (NSS) is the preferred solution used during blood transfusions.

Colloids

Colloids are substances that have a higher molecular weight than crystalloids and therefore cannot pass through the vascular membrane. Colloids increase intravascular fluid volume. When colloid therapy is used, less fluid is needed to reestablish the fluid volume in the vascular space. Table 17-8 lists the colloids that may be used for fluid replacement.

The colloids albumin 5%, plasma protein fraction (Plasmanate), and hetastarch increase the vascular volume to approximately the same amount that is infused. With low-molecular-weight dextran 40, the vascular fluid is expanded by one to two times the amount that is infused. With albumin 25%, the vascular volume is expanded four times the amount that is infused.

Crystalloids, Colloids, and Blood Products

Crystalloids are the first choice for treating hypovolemic shock. Crystalloids can restore fluid volume in the vascular and interstitial spaces and improve renal function; however, large quantities of crystalloids are needed. Excessive infusions of crystalloids might cause fluid overload in clients who are elderly or who have heart disease. Frequently, a combination of crystalloids and colloids is used for fluid replacement. If severe blood loss occurs, blood transfusions may be necessary after infusion of

Table 17-8

Colloids

Colloids*	Brand Names	Comments
Blood products	Packed RBCs Whole blood	Used to replace blood loss.
Albumin, 5% or 25%	Albuminar Plasbumin	Not used in acute shock; 1–4 mL/min.
Plasma protein fraction, 5%	Plasmanate	Rapid infusion rate can decrease blood pressure.
Hetastarch	Hespan	Synthetic starch similar to human glycogen. Very expensive.
Dextran 40	Dextran	Low-molecular-weight dextran 40 may prolong bleeding time.

*Colloid therapy is more expensive than crystalloid therapy.

1 to 2 L of crystalloids. Each fluid replacement situation differs and each individual situation must be evaluated separately.

There are suggested formulas for restoring fluid loss, especially for clients in hypovolemic shock who have had some blood loss, moderate blood loss, or massive amounts of blood and body fluid loss. The simplest formula for fluid replacement is the 3:1 rule; for every 1 mL of blood lost, 3 mL of crystalloid solution are necessary to restore fluid volume. If hypotension persists despite 2 L of crystalloid solution replacement, a blood transfusion should be considered. When administering normal saline solution (NSS) or lactated Ringer's solution for hypovolemic shock, the IV solutions may be given rapidly at first to decrease the symptoms of shock and prevent a fluid shift into the interstitial space at the injured site. Later, the flow rate should be slowed. Table 17-9 lists the four classes of hypovolemic shock with their estimated amount of blood loss and percent of blood volume loss (% BV), changes in vital signs, pulse pressure, urine output, and types of fluid replacement.

Vasopressors

Many years ago the first and foremost treatment of shock was to administer a vasopressor drug. The drug constricts the dilated blood vessels that occur with shock and raises the blood pressure. Vasopressors act as a temporary treatment for shock; if the cause of the shock is not alleviated, the progress of shock increases. Today, vasopressors are only used

Table 17-9

Classes of Hypovolemic Shock and Appropriate Fluid Replacement

Characteristic Effects of Hypovolemic Shock	Class I Mild Shock	Class II Moderate Shock	Class III Severe Shock	Class IV Severe Shock
Blood loss	<750 mL or 1½ units	750–1500 mL or 1½–3 units	1500–2000 mL or 3–4 units	>2000 mL or >4 units
Blood loss (% BV)	<15%	15–30%	30–40%	>40%
Heart rate (bpm)	<100	>100	>120	>140
Blood pressure	Normal	Normal to slightly decreased	Decreased	Decreased
Pulse pressure	Normal or increased	Decreased from normal	Decreased 20–25 mm Hg	Decreased 20 mm Hg or less
Urine output	>30 mL/h	20–30 mL/h	5–15 mL/h	0–5 mL/h
Fluid replacement (3:1 rule) 3 mL replaced for 1 mL of blood loss	Crystalloid: NSS or lactated Ringer's	Crystalloid: NSS or lactated Ringer's	Crystalloid and blood	Crystalloid and blood

for severe shock or types of shock that do not respond to treatment. Note that vasopressors are *not* effective in the treatment of hypovolemic shock because constricting the blood vessels does not aid in the circulation of blood when the cause is most obvious, a lack of blood. Replacing blood volume loss should correct this type of shock. Table 17-10 outlines the clinical management for alleviating four types of clinical shock: hypovolemic, cardiogenic, septic, and neurogenic.

When vasopressors are used, cardiac dysrhythmias may occur. Levarterenol bitartrate (Levophed) is norepinephrine, which is a strong vasopressor. It increases the blood pressure and cardiac output by constricting blood vessels. Epinephrine works in the same manner. Dopamine HCl (Intropin) is a catecholamine precursor of norepinephrine. It increases blood pressure and cardiac output. It also dilates renal vessels at a low dose, thus increasing renal blood flow and the glomerular filtration rate. Levophed causes vasoconstriction, which affects the renal

Table 17-10

Clinical Management of Shock States

Hypovolemic Shock	Cardiogenic Shock	Septic Shock	Neurogenic Shock
1. O_2	1. O_2	1. O_2	1. O_2

2. IV fluids, such as
  a. Lactated Ringer's
  b. Normal saline
  c. Blood products
	2. IV therapy is limited when pulmonary congestion is present and venous pressure is elevated. Close monitoring of CVP and PCWP	2. IV therapy crystalloids	2. IV therapy

3. No vasopressors		3. Vasopressors for nonresponsiveness	3. Vasopressors, if necessary
4. Electrolyte replacement	3. Vasopressors, if necessary	4. Blood cultures	4. Atropine for symptomatic bradycardia
	4. Antiarrythmics Sodium nitroprusside/ Nipride, nitroglycerin/NTG; (decrease preload and decrease afterload). Intropic drugs (e.g., dobutamine/Dobutrex, amrinone/Inocor) Sedatives Diuretics	5. IV antibiotics	

Note: Examples of vasopressors are (1) levarterenol bitartrate/Levophed, (2) dopamine hydrochloride/Intropin, (3) epinephrine infusion.

arteries and can decrease renal function. Vasopressors are titrated according to the blood pressure and should be checked every 2 to 5 minutes. Dobutamine (Dobutrex) is an adrenergic drug that moderately increases blood pressure by increasing the heart rate and cardiac output. Dobutamine is effective in increasing myocardial contractility.

● Clinical Considerations: Trauma and Shock

1. In trauma and shock, check for signs and symptoms that may indicate hypovolemia and shock, such as restlessness, apprehension, confusion, tachycardia, narrowing of the pulse pressure (20 mm Hg or less), tachypnea, and cool and clammy skin.

2. Urinary output may be decreased. Report if urine output is less than 25 mL per hour or 200 mL per 8 hours. If the serum creatinine is elevated, renal dysfunction may be present due to a lack of renal perfusion related to shock.

3. Recognize that the hemoglobin, hematocrit, and BUN may be elevated during a hypovolemic state. With a large amount of blood loss, the hemoglobin drops, but not immediately.

4. Monitor intravenous therapy. The choice crystalloids are normal saline solution (NSS) and lactated Ringer's solution. Five percent dextrose and water should not be used to correct hypovolemia during shock.

5. Crystalloids are usually administered rapidly during early shock to increase blood pressure, hydrate the client, and increase urine output. Check for fluid overload in the young, elderly, and debilitated person. Signs and symptoms of overhydration are chest rales, constant irritated cough, neck and/or hand vein engorgement, and dyspnea.

6. A simple formula for fluid replacement is the 3:1 rule; for every 1 mL of blood loss, 3 mL of crystalloid solution are needed to restore fluid volume. If hypotension persists despite 2 L of rapidly administered crystalloid solutions, blood transfusion is probably needed.

7. Colloids are used to treat shock when less fluid is needed.

8. Vasopressors are seldom used except to treat progressive shock and nonresponsive treatment to shock. Dopamine is the vasopressor of choice because it does not affect renal arteries at a low dose. Other vasopressors cause vasoconstriction, thus decreasing blood flow to the kidneys and decreasing renal function.

9. Metabolic acidosis (lactic acidosis) frequently results from cellular damage and lack of fluid and nutrients to cells associated with severe hypovolemia and shock. In acidosis, the pH is below 7.35, HCO_3 is below 24 mEq/L, and base excess (BE) is less than -2.

❱ CLIENT MANAGEMENT

Assessment

- Check vital signs and report signs and symptoms that may indicate hypovolemia and shock, such as tachycardia, narrowing of the pulse pressure (20 mm Hg or less is an indicator of shock), tachypnea, and cool, clammy skin.

- Obtain a drug history. Report if the client is taking insulin, potassium-wasting diuretics, digoxin, steroid preparations, beta blockers, or calcium channel blockers.

- Assess the behavioral and neurologic status of the injured client and/or the client in shock. Irritability, apprehension, restlessness, and confusion are symptoms of a fluid volume deficit. Apprehension and restlessness are early symptoms of shock.

- Check urinary output. Less than 25 mL per hour or 200 mL per 8 hours may indicate fluid volume deficit or renal insufficiency. In severe shock, severe oliguria or anuria may occur.

- Check laboratory results, especially hemoglobin, hematocrit, arterial blood gases (ABG), serum electrolytes, BUN, and serum creatinine. Report abnormal findings.

Diagnoses

- Fluid volume deficit, related to traumatic injury and shock.
- Fluid volume excess, related to massive infusions of crystalloids.
- Altered tissue perfusion (renal, cardiopulmonary, cerebral, and peripheral), related to decreased blood volume and circulation secondary to hypovolemia and shock.
- Altered urinary elimination less than body requirement, related to fluid volume deficit and shock.

Interventions

- Monitor vital signs. Compare the vital signs with those taken on admission and report differences immediately.

- Check skin color and turgor. Note changes; pallor; gray, cold, clammy skin; and poor skin turgor are symptoms of shock and fluid volume deficit.

- Monitor IV therapy. Crystalloids are usually administered rapidly initially to hydrate the client, increase blood pressure, and increase urine output. Normal saline solution (NSS) and lactated Ringer's solution are the crystalloids of choice.

- Auscultate the lungs for rales. Overhydration from excessive fluids and rapid administration of IV fluids can cause pulmonary edema.

- Check for neck vein engorgement when overhydration is suspected.

- Check for pitting edema in the feet and legs. Weigh the client daily to determine if there is fluid retention.

- Monitor central venous pressure (CVP) and pulmonary capillary wedge pressure (PCWP), which are needed to adjust fluid balance. The norm for CVP is 5–12 cm/H_2O or 2–4 mm Hg (+ to −2), and for PCWP is 4–12 mm Hg. Keeping PCWP between 12 and 15 mm Hg in shock conditions provides the filling pressure required for adequate stroke volume and cardiac output. If PCWP drops below 10 mm Hg, administration of fluid is usually needed. If PCWP is greater than 18 mm HG, fluid restriction may be necessary.

- Monitor urine output. Hourly urine should be measured and if less than 25 mL/h, the IV fluid rate should be increased as ordered. Do not forget to check for overhydration when pushing fluids, IV or orally.

- Report systolic blood pressure of 80 mm Hg or less immediately. Kidney damage can occur due to poor renal perfusion during hypotensive states.

- Monitor laboratory results. Compare laboratory test results with those taken on admission.

- Monitor ECG readings and report arrhythmias (ST–T changes), which may be indicative of a potassium imbalance or cardiac ischemia.

- Monitor arterial blood gases (ABG). Metabolic acidosis frequently results from cellular damage due to severe hypovolemia and shock. In acidosis, the pH is below 7.35, HCO_3 is below 24 mEq/L, and base excess (BE) is less than -2. Respiratory acidosis may also result due to the lungs' inability to excrete carbon dioxide.

Evaluation/Outcome

- Evaluate whether the cause of the shock has been controlled or eliminated.

- Verify that the client remains free of shocklike symptoms.

- Evaluate that the urine output is within normal range (600 to 1400 mL/per 24 hours).

- Evaluate the effects of IV therapy in controlling or alleviating shock.

- Determine that the laboratory results are within normal ranges.

Gastrointestinal Surgical Interventions

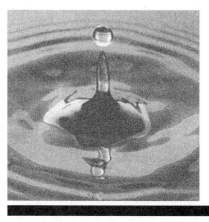

▶ INTRODUCTION

Fluid and electrolyte changes may occur in a client following a surgical procedure. Surgical interventions geared to correct gastrointestinal problems put the client at greater risk for fluid and electrolyte disturbances than other types of surgical procedures. Diagnostic testing and preparation for gastrointestinal (GI) surgery may further increase the client's risk for fluid, electrolyte, and acid-base imbalances. Postoperatively, the client may be NPO (nothing by mouth), have a gastrointestinal drainage tube, and have delayed peristalsis, which further contribute to the imbalances. Preexisting cardiopulmonary, endocrine, and renal conditions in conjunction with the use of diuretics, glucocorticoids, and insulin place the client undergoing GI surgery at a high risk for fluid, electrolyte, and acid-base imbalances. Assessment of these imbalances must begin preoperatively and continue postoperatively. Alterations in fluid volume status can occur rapidly; thus, astute assessment skills and timely interventions are essential to prevent or decrease potential complications.

▶ ELECTROLYTE CONCENTRATION IN THE GASTROINTESTINAL TRACT

Electrolytes are most plentiful in the gastrointestinal tract. The concentration of sodium, potassium, and bicarbonate ions is higher in the intestines than in the stomach. Chloride ion concentration is approximately the same in the intestines and stomach. However, the hydrogen ion is in higher concentration in the stomach and the bicarbonate ion concentration is higher in the intestines. A decrease in the number of hydrogen ions in the stomach can cause metabolic alkalosis, while a loss of the number of bicarbonate ions in the intestines can result in metabolic acidosis. Table 18-1 lists the concentrations of electrolytes in the stomach and intestine.

▶ PATHOPHYSIOLOGY, ETIOLOGY, AND CLINICAL MANIFESTATIONS RELATED TO GI PROBLEMS

Clients undergoing a minor surgical procedure usually do not experience fluid, electrolyte, and/or acid-base disturbances. Following a major surgical procedure, sodium and water may be retained and potassium may be lost. Many clients undergoing gastrointestinal surgery experience fluid and electrolyte imbalances prior to surgery that often put them in a debilitated state. Vomiting and/or diarrhea are common conditions that may indicate a gastrointestinal problem that calls for surgical intervention. When fluids are lost, important electrolytes such as sodium, chloride, potassium, bicarbonate (intestine), and hydrogen (stomach) are also lost. Treatment of these fluid and electrolyte imbalances must be

Table 18-1

Concentration of Electrolytes in the Stomach and Intestine (mEq/L)

Area	Body Fluid	Na^+	K^+	Cl^-	HCO_3^-	
Stomach	Gastric juice	60.4	9.2	100*	0–14	H^+*
Small intestine	Intestinal juice	111.3*	20*	104.2*	31*	

*Electrolytes that are highly concentrated in these areas.

considered both prior to surgery and in conjunction with the concurrent fluid losses during the procedure. Replacement of fluid and electrolyte losses is necessary before, during, and following surgery.

If a severe fluid volume deficit results from prolonged vomiting and/or diarrhea, urine output is decreased, and tachycardia and postural hypotension occur. The fluid loss results in a hemoconcentration, causing the hemoglobin, hematocrit, and BUN levels to rise. Fluid balance and adequate urine output need to be restored prior to surgery. If a gastric tube is inserted prior to surgery to prevent vomiting, fluid and electrolytes are lost through GI suctioning. Serum sodium and potassium levels may be decreased, normal, or elevated. The sodium, chloride, and potassium are lost because of vomiting, diarrhea, or GI suctioning; however, if the fluid volume deficit is severe, the hemoconcentration causes elevated serum electrolyte levels. With GI disturbances, hydrogen and chloride ions are lost from the gastric juices, resulting in metabolic alkalosis. Frequently, potassium is also lost, so the imbalance is hypokalemic alkalosis. Table 18-2 lists the causes, pathophysiologic changes, and clinical manifestations related to GI disturbances.

Table 18-2

Pathophysiologic Changes, Etiology, and Clinical Manifestations Related to Gastrointestinal Problems Prior to Surgery

Etiology	Pathophysiologic Changes	Clinical Manifestations
Vomiting/diarrhea	ECF and ICF loss Electrolyte loss (sodium, chloride, potassium, and hydrogen or bicarbonate) Acid-base imbalance (if severe) Hypokalemic alkalosis: loss of hydrogen and potassium from stomach Metabolic acidosis: loss of bicarbonate from intestines	Tachycardia Postural hypotension Dry mucous membrane Decreased skin turgor Decreased urine output *Laboratory Changes* ↑ Hemoglobin ↑ Hematocrit ↑ BUN ↓, Normal, ↑ Sodium ↓, ↑ Potassium ↓ Bicarbonate (diarrhea)
Gastric suction	Prolonged GI suctioning: similar to vomiting	Laboratory changes similar to vomiting

▶ CLINICAL MANAGEMENT

Clinical management of fluid, electrolyte, and acid-base imbalances for GI surgical clients can occur both preoperatively and postoperatively. Preoperative and postoperative management are addressed separately here.

Preoperative Management

Clients who are vomiting, have diarrhea, or are receiving gastric suctioning should be assessed for fluid and electrolyte imbalances. Fluid and electrolyte replacements are necessary prior to surgery to restore balance and maintain adequate urine output. Once signs, symptoms, and laboratory changes related to fluid and electrolyte imbalances are noted, immediate replacements for these imbalances are essential. Correction of imbalances and proper maintenance of body fluids and electrolytes decreases complications and promotes a speedy recovery period.

In healthy preoperative clients, long periods of being NPO prior to surgery are unnecessary. The usual is NPO after midnight prior to surgery. This is to avoid nausea and vomiting resulting from the anesthesia. With today's anesthetics, this is not a common problem. No solid foods should be taken after midnight; however, clear liquids may be taken up to 3 hours before surgery depending on the type of surgery and the policies of the health professional team.

Postoperative Management

During surgery fluid loss due to bleeding and/or shifting of intravascular fluid to the surgical site (third-space fluid) can cause a decrease in the volume of circulating vascular fluid. A balanced electrolyte (salt) solution such as lactated Ringer's is usually administered during the intraoperative period and a blood transfusion may be administered if the blood loss is 500 to 1000 mL and the client's vital signs and health status require replacement. Central venous pressure is monitored during the operative procedure in high-risk clients to determine fluid replacement.

Surgical procedures, anesthesia, trauma, and pain contribute to an increased release of the antidiuretic hormone (ADH). Excessive release of ADH is called the syndrome of inappropriate ADH or SIADH. Excess ADH release may persist for 12 to 24 hours after surgery. This causes fluid to be reabsorbed from the renal tubules and decreased urine output. Surgical procedures can also promote the increased secretion of aldosterone, resulting in sodium and fluid retention and potassium loss. Elderly and young children experiencing gastrointestinal surgical interventions are at the highest risk for the neuroendocrine response (ADH and aldosterone).

Gastric or intestinal intubation (tube passed into the stomach or intestines for suctioning purposes) is often performed before surgery. This alleviates vomiting due to an obstruction in the gastrointestinal tract or decompresses the stomach or bowel, or both, before and after the operative procedure.

Following abdominal surgery, a gastric or an intestinal tube is frequently inserted to remove secretions until peristalsis returns and to relieve abdominal distention. For gastric intubation, a Levine tube or Salem sump is inserted via the nose into the stomach. For an intestinal intubation, a Miller-Abbott tube or Cantor tube is inserted via the nose to the stomach and into the intestines. Intestinal tubes are longer than gastric tubes and they contain a small balloon filled with air or mercury that helps the tube move into the lower intestines. Urine output should be at least 25 mL/h and preferably 30 to 50 mL/h. Three liters or more of intravenous balanced salt solution are usually administered during the first 24 hours for fluid loss. Electrolytes are replaced according to the serum electrolyte levels.

Solid particles may accumulate and obstruct the gastrointestinal tubing. Irrigating the tube assures patency and proper drainage. Frequent irrigations using large amounts of water should be avoided to prevent electrolyte washout. Gastric tubes are irrigated at specific intervals with small amounts of normal saline solution to prevent electrolyte loss. Sometimes small amounts of air are ordered to check the patency of the tube instead of irrigating the tube with saline. Listen with the stethoscope over the stomach for a "whoosh" sound when air is injected to confirm the patency of the tube. Because suction removes fluids and electrolytes, oral fluid intake is restricted and parenteral therapy is initiated. Sips of water can alleviate the dryness in the mouth and lessen irritation in the throat, if allowed. However, one must be cautioned that water dilutes the electrolytes in the stomach and the suction then removes them.

A feeling of fullness, vomiting, and abdominal distention are signs and symptoms that peristalsis has not returned. Checking periodically for bowel sounds is necessary to determine when peristalsis has returned.

An H_2 receptor antagonist (H_2 blocker) such as cimetidine (Tagamet), ranitidine (Zantac), or famotidine (Pepcid) is commonly administered to clients through the gastric tube. This group of drugs suppresses hydrochloric acid (HCl) production, thus minimizing the amount of HCl removed by gastric suction.

Coughing and deep breathing help to keep the lungs inflated and promote effective gas exchange. Inadequate ventilation due to pain, narcotics, and anesthesia causes alveolar collapse and eventually leads to CO_2 retention (respiratory acidosis). Table 18-3 lists the clinical management for clients following GI surgery.

Table 18-3

Clinical Management for Pre- and Postoperative GI Surgery

Clinical Management	Rationale
Preoperative	
Fluid balance	Replace fluid loss. Three to five liters of balanced electrolyte solution (BES) may be necessary prior to surgery.
Electrolyte balance	Replace sodium and potassium as indicated by the serum electrolyte levels.
Urine output	Hourly urine output should be monitored. Urine output should be at least 25 mL/h and preferably 30 to 50 mL/h.
Postoperative	
Fluid balance	Serum osmolality should be between 280 to 295 mOsm/kg. To determine serum osmolality, use the formula: $$2 \times \text{Serum sodium} + \frac{\text{BUN}}{3} + \frac{\text{Glucose}}{18} = \text{Serum osmolality}$$ A decreased serum osmolality may indicate hemodilution and an elevated serum osmolality indicates hemoconcentration. At least 3 liters of BES daily is indicated. Check for overhydration if the IV solution runs too fast.
Gastric or intestinal intubation	GI tubing should be patent. Plain water should not be used to maintain patency of tube; electrolytes are "washed out." Small amounts of saline solution or air may be indicated to maintain tube patency.
Electrolyte balance	Sodium and potassium gains or losses can be determined by periodically checking the serum electrolyte levels. Signs and symptoms of electrolyte imbalance should be reported.
Acid-base balance	Deep breathing and coughing improve gas exchange and prevent CO_2 retention and respiratory acidosis. Metabolic alkalosis may result from gastric suctioning because of the loss of the hydrogen and chloride ions (hydrochloric acid).
Peristalsis	Bowel sounds in the four quadrants should be checked to determine if peristalsis has returned. The gastrointestinal tube is usually removed when peristalsis has returned.
Medications H$_2$ blockers	Cimetidine, ranitidine, or famotidine suppresses the production of hydrochloric acid. The amount of HCl removed by gastric suction is diminished.

● Clinical Considerations: Gastrointestinal Surgical Intervention

1. Check for fluid and electrolyte imbalances prior to any type of surgery, especially gastrointestinal surgery. Indicators of fluid volume deficit are tachycardia, postural hypotension, dry mucous membranes, and poor skin turgor.

2. Monitor urinary output per hour, every 8 hours, and per day prior to and following surgery. Urine output may be decreased prior to surgery due to fluid volume deficit and may decrease following surgery because of SIADH.

3. Check laboratory test results for fluid volume deficit (FVD), i.e., increased hemoglobin, increased hematocrit, increased BUN (all caused by hemoconcentration), and decreased serum potassium level, decreased/normal/elevated serum sodium level, decreased serum bicarbonate level (due to intestinal involvement).

4. Loss of hydrogen and chloride ions (hydrochloric acid) from gastric secretions causes metabolic alkalosis. Loss of bicarbonate from the intestinal secretions may cause metabolic acidosis.

5. The stomach and intestines are rich in electrolytes, especially sodium, chloride, potassium, hydrogen (stomach), and bicarbonate (intestine).

6. Intravenous fluid replacements for fluid volume deficits are balanced electrolyte solutions (BES) such as lactated Ringer's or normal saline solution (0.9% NaCl).

7. Avoid administering 5% dextrose and water continuously. This isotonic IV solution becomes hypotonic when dextrose is rapidly metabolized leaving only the water, which dilutes the electrolyte levels.

8. Following abdominal surgery, peristalsis is decreased or absent. GI intubation is usually prescribed. Bowel sounds should be monitored to determine the presence of peristalsis.

▶ CLIENT MANAGEMENT

Assessment

- Prior to gastrointestinal surgery, assess for preexisting health problems and medications that can further increase the potential risk for fluid and electrolyte disturbances. Uncorrected preoperative hypovolemia and anemia may increase the risk for fluid and electrolyte disturbances postoperatively.

- Check the vital signs and use the results as a baseline for future comparisons. A fluid volume deficit may cause tachycardia, postural or orthostatic hypotension, and a decreased pulse pressure.
- Check intake, output, and weight. Urine output may decrease during a fluid volume deficit.
- Assess client's bowel sounds. Note if peristalsis is present prior to surgery.
- Assess for fluid volume deficit. Check serum osmolality; FVD is present if the level is elevated.
- Check laboratory test results. Note if hemoglobin, hematocrit, and BUN are elevated; these are indicators of a fluid volume deficit.
- If a gastric tube is inserted, check that the tube is draining.

Diagnoses

- Fluid volume deficit, related to gastrointestinal loss, decreased fluid intake, and/or fluid volume shift.
- Pain, related to trauma from abdominal surgery.
- Impaired tissue integrity, related to surgery, decreased or absence of bowel sounds, and decreased GI motility (peristalsis).
- Ineffective airway clearance, related to pain, ineffective coughing, deep breathing, and viscous mucous secretions.
- Altered urinary elimination, related to fluid volume deficit secondary to gastrointestinal disturbance.

Interventions

- Monitor vital signs every 4 hours or more frequently if the client is unstable. Hypovolemia causes reflex tachycardia and postural hypotension.
- Check mucous membranes and skin turgor. Poor skin turgor with dry, scaly skin and dry mucous membranes indicate a fluid volume deficit.
- Monitor urinary output. Report if the output is less than 600 mL per day. Urine output of 750 mL plus per day is preferable.
- Monitor laboratory results. Note if the hemoglobin, hematocrit, and BUN are elevated, which is indicative of hemocentration resulting from fluid volume deficit.

- Monitor serum electrolyte results. Serum potassium is usually decreased because of FVD; however, potassium may be increased because of hemoconcentration due to FVD.

- Encourage coughing and deep breathing to improve alveolar expansion and mobilize secretions.

- Monitor intravenous flow rate. IV solutions that run too fast or a health status that does not warrant a large volume of fluids may cause the client to develop a fluid overload or overhydration.

- Monitor bowel sounds to determine the return of peristalsis.

- Check that the gastrointestinal tube is patent. Irrigate with normal saline solution or air according to the order.

Evaluation/Outcome

- Evaluate that the source of the ECFV problem has been eliminated or controlled.

- Evaluate the effectiveness of interventions (fluid and electrolyte replacement therapy, gastrointestinal intubation, medications, pain control measures, and so on) in balancing fluid needs and promoting comfort.

- Determine that the laboratory test results are within normal range.

- Monitor vital signs (particularly blood pressure and pulse rate) for stability.

- Evaluate renal function. Urine output is adequate and within normal volume.

CHAPTER 19

Chronic Diseases with Fluid and Electrolyte Imbalances: Heart Failure, Diabetic Ketoacidosis, and Chronic Obstructive Pulmonary Disease

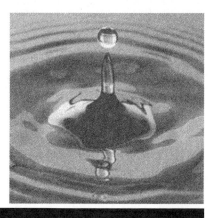

❱ INTRODUCTION

A chronic disease, as defined by the U.S. National Center for Health Statistics, is a chronic condition that has a duration of 3 months or longer. Chronic conditions usually progress slowly over a long period of time. Chronic illnesses frequently do not occur as a single health problem, but are associated with multiple chronic health problems, e.g., a person with uncontrolled diabetes mellitus or chronic obstructive pulmonary disease (COPD) often develops heart failure (HF). This chapter addresses three common chronic diseases: (1) congestive heart failure (CHF), (2) diabetes mellitus (ketoacidosis), and (3) chronic obstructive pulmonary disease (COPD).

❱ CONGESTIVE HEART FAILURE (CHF)

CHF is a chronic disease process secondary to major disease entities, i.e., long-time diabetes mellitus, coronary heart disease, hypertension, pulmonary diseases, kidney diseases, and hyperthyroidism. Congestive heart failure is a type of heart failure characterized by an inability of the heart to pump an adequate supply of blood (pump failure) to meet the needs of tissue perfusion. CHF is circulatory congestion related to pump failure. It develops slowly, begins with milder symptoms, and usually does not become severe until compensatory mechanisms fail.

Pathophysiology

CHF is primarily characterized by left ventricular failure to pump sufficient blood to the body tissues and cells. Failure of the left ventricle frequently leads to failure of the right ventricle. Blood does not circulate efficiently, but "pools" in the intravascular system. Clients with cardiomyopathy usually have failure of both ventricles, thus displaying signs and symptoms of pulmonary edema and peripheral edema. CHF is often secondary to other major disease entities. Table 19-1 lists the pathophysiologic factors associated with CHF and the compensatory mechanisms to prevent heart failure. Left-sided and right-sided heart failures present different symptoms.

In early heart failure, the heart compensates via ventricular dilatation, ventricular hypertrophy, and tachycardia in order to meet oxygen, nutrient, and circulatory needs. The ventricle enlarges to increase output and circulation; however, when the ventricle dilates, the heart needs more oxygen. Ventricular hypertrophy causes the ventricle wall to thicken and increases heart contractility. Increased heart rate increases circulation, but when the heart rate is too rapid, the ventricles are unable to fill adequately. When there is failure of the three compensatory mechanisms to maintain heart function, cardiac decompensation occurs, resulting in pulmonary edema (left-sided heart failure) and/or peripheral edema (right-sided heart failure).

Etiology

Reasons that the heart fails include: (1) increased preload due to increased blood volume, (2) increased afterload because of increased pump resistance, and (3) decreased heart contractility. Causes of increased preload are mitral and/or aortic regurgitation, and ventricular septal defects. Aortic stenosis and systemic hypertension cause pump resistance or increased afterload. Myocardial infarction and cardiomyopathy can cause decreased heart contractility. Table 19-2 lists the causes of left and right heart failure.

Table 19-1

Pathophysiologic Changes Associated With CHF

Pathophysiologic Changes	Rationale
Cardiac reserve (decreased) ↓	Decreased cardiac reserve is the inability of the heart to respond to increased burden, e.g., fever, exercise, or excitement.
Cardiac compensation	The heart, in early heart failure, compensates for loss of cardiac reserve. Over an extended period of time the heart increases its cardiac output through ventricular dilatation, ventricular hypertrophy, and tachycardia.
Ventricular dilatation	Muscle fibers of the myocardium increase in length and the ventricle enlarges to augment its output. Heart muscle stretches to a certain point and then ceases to increase heart contractility. A dilated heart needs more oxygen than a "normal" heart; however, the decreased coronary blood flow limits the O_2 supply to the heart muscle.
Ventricular hypertrophy	There is increased thickening of the ventricular wall, which increases the weight of the heart. Ventricular hypertrophy mostly follows dilatation, and hypertrophy aids in heart contractility. A hypertrophied heart works harder than a normal heart and has a greater O_2 need.
Tachycardia	The increased heart rate is the least effective of the three compensatory mechanisms. The heart rate increases to a point that the ventricles are unable to fill adequately. As the heart rate increases, diastole time is reduced. The stroke volume first decreases, causing the cardiac output to increase, and later decreases as the heart rate greatly increases and diastole time shortens.
Cardiac decompensation	Occurs when the three compensatory mechanisms fail to maintain heart function and adequate circulation. Symptoms begin to develop with normal activity.
Left-sided heart failure	Generally results from left ventricular damage to the myocardium. The heart is at first unable to eject the full blood volume from the ventricle. Three compensatory mechanisms come into play. With compensatory mechanism failure, residual blood remains in the dilated ventricle. The left atrium dilates and atrial hypertrophy results. When the atrium is unable to receive blood from pulmonary veins, pulmonary congestion or pulmonary edema occurs. Etiologic factors include hypertension, myocardial infarction (heart attack), rheumatic fever affecting aortic valve, and syphilis. Symptoms of left-sided heart failure are similar to symptoms of overhydration, i.e., irritated cough, dizziness, engorged neck veins, moist rales.
Right-sided heart failure	Generally results from increased pressure in the pulmonary vascular system. The right ventricle tries to pump blood into the congested lungs, thus meeting resistance. Blood and fluids "back up" into the venous circulation, causing congestion in the GI tract, liver, and kidneys. Peripheral edema also occurs. Right-sided heart failure generally follows left-sided heart failure; however, occasionally, it is independent of left-sided failure. Symptoms of right-sided heart failure include liver congestion and enlargement, fullness in abdomen, and peripheral edema of lower extremities, mostly refractory and pitting.

Table 19-2

Etiology of Congestive Heart Failure

Factors Affecting Heart Failure	Causes
Left-Sided Heart Failure	
Increased preload	Mitral regurgitation
	Aortic regurgitation
	Ventricular septal defects
	Hypervolemia
Increased afterload	Systemic hypertension
	Aortic stenosis
	Hypertrophic cardiomyopathy
Myocardial dysfunction	Myocardial infarction
	Myocarditis
	Cardiomyopathy
	Coronary artery disease
	Dysrhythmias
Right-Sided Heart Failure	Pulmonary hypertension
	Left ventricular failure
	Myocardial infarction (right ventricular area)

Clinical Manifestations

The heart compensates for inadequate blood flow by increasing the heart rate; thus, the blood pressure and respirations increase. The respiratory rate increases to improve the oxygen intake. Table 19-3 lists the clinical manifestations with rationales associated with CHF. As the compensatory mechanisms fail to adequately control, left-sided ventricular failure and/or pulmonary edema occurs, resulting in signs and symptoms similar to ECFVE or overhydration (constant irritated cough, chest rales, neck vein engorgement, and dyspnea). Right-sided heart failure may also result. Symptoms include pitting edema in the extremities. Serum sodium and potassium levels may be normal or low due to hemodilution related to an excess of extracellular fluid. The serum osmolality may also reflect a low normal reading or decreased reading due to the ECFVE.

Clinical Management

The first line of management for CHF is the "three Ds," diet, a digitalis preparation, and diuretics. A low sodium diet is usually prescribed and fluid intake is limited to 1200 mL or less. Digoxin is given for the first

Table 19-3

Clinical Manifestations Associated with CHF

Clinical Manifestations	Rationale
Vital Signs (VS)	
Increased pulse rate (tachycardia)	Increased heart rate is a compensatory mechanism to improve circulation of the blood.
Increased respiration (tachypnea)	Respirations increase to increase oxygen intake for tissue oxygenation.
Increased blood pressure (hypertension)	When hypertension occurs, it is usually because of atherosclerosis. Noncirculating vascular fluid can also increase blood pressure.
Edema	
Pulmonary	Caused by left-sided heart failure. (Because of pump failure, fluid "backs up" in the pulmonary system, causing fluid congestion in the lung tissues.) Fluid inhibits adequate gas exchange (O_2 and CO_2). Signs and symptoms of pulmonary edema are similar to the signs and symptoms of overhydration.
Peripheral	May result from right-sided heart failure. Fluids accumulate in the extremities due to the fluid back-up in the venous circulation.
Cyanosis	Cyanosis is a sign of hypoxia due to inadequate blood flow to body tissues.
Laboratory Results	
Plasma/serum sodium: increased (hypernatremia) or normal	Sodium retention in the extracellular fluid (ECF) usually occurs even when the serum sodium is within normal range or lower. Hemodilution can cause a normal or slightly lower serum sodium level.
Plasma/serum potassium: normal or decreased (hypokalemia)	The serum potassium level can be decreased with the use of potassium-wasting diuretics and due to hemodilution from fluid volume excess.
Plasma/serum magnesium: normal or decreased (hypomagnesemia)	Long-term use of potassium-wasting diuretics can cause both hypomagnesemia and hypokalemia.
Serum osmolality: < 280 mOsm/kg	Due to hemodilution. If the serum sodium level is increased, the serum osmolality increases.

day or more in loading doses. Digoxin has a half-life of 36 hours, so digitalization (increased doses of digoxin) is needed to achieve a desired physiologic response. Digoxin is a cardiac glycoside (cardiotonic), which slows the ventricular contractions and increases the forcefulness of the contractions, thus increasing cardiac output. Diuretics are used to excrete sodium and water. Furosemide (Lasix) is a diuretic commonly administered intravenously and orally. This diuretic (a potassium-wasting diuretic) not only excretes sodium, but excretes potassium, calcium, and magnesium as well. When the serum potassium level decreases because of the use of potent potassium-wasting diuretics, ventricular dysrhythmias result from hypokalemia (K <3.2 mEq/L). Serum potassium and sodium levels need to be closely monitored. Serum digoxin levels have a narrow therapeutic range (0.5–2.0 mg/mL).

Other drug therapy used to control CHF includes beta-adrenergic agonists, phosphodiesterase inhibitors, angiotensin-converting enzyme (ACE) inhibitors, and vasodilators. Both beta-adrenergic agonists and ACE inhibitors increase cardiac output. Cardiac glycosides, sympathomimetics (beta-adrenergic agonists), and phosphodiesterase (PDE) inhibitors are three positive inotropic group agents that exert an effect on the heart by increasing myocardial contractility. Table 19-4 lists the drug categories and doses used to manage CHF.

● Clinical Considerations: Congestive Heart Failure (CHF)

1. Knowledge of the signs and symptoms of left-sided heart failure and right-sided heart failure. With left-sided heart failure (pulmonary edema), check for chest rales, dyspnea, constant irritated cough, and neck vein engorgement. With right-sided failure (peripheral edema), check for pitting edema in the extremities in the morning before the client rises.

2. For quick assessment of overhydration because of heart failure, check for hand vein engorgement. Lower the hand below the heart level until the hand veins are engorged; then raise the hand above the heart level. If the hand veins remain engorged above the heart level for 10 to 15 seconds, fluid volume excess is likely to be present.

3. Serum sodium and potassium should be monitored. If the client is taking digoxin and a potassium-wasting diuretic such as furosemide (Lasix), daily potassium supplements should be administered. If the client is taking digoxin and furosemide or hydrochlorothiazide, hypokalemia (serum potassium loss) is likely to occur. Hypokalemia enhances the action of digoxin and can cause digitalis toxicity (slow, irregular pulse, anorexia, nausea, vomiting, and visual disturbances).

4. Check for signs and symptoms of hypokalemia; e.g., dizziness, muscular weakness, abdominal distention, diminished peristalsis, and dysrhythmia.

Table 19-4

Medications for the Control of CHF

Drug	Rationale
Digitalis Preparation Digoxin	Digoxin exerts a positive inotropic action on the heart, increasing the contractility of the myocardium. To increase the blood level of digoxin when first used, a digitalization program over 24 hours is prescribed; e.g., 1.0–1.5 mg dose divided over 24 hours, then maintenance doses of 0.125–0.25 mg are prescribed daily. A serum digoxin level of >2.0 mg/mL causes digitalis toxicity; therefore, the serum level needs to be closely monitored. Signs and symptoms of digitalis toxicity include anorexia, nausea, vomiting, diarrhea, bradycardia (pulse rate <60), and visual disturbances.
Diuretics **Loop or High-Ceiling** Furosemide (Lasix)	Diuretics increase urine output, which decreases fluid volume. A loop diuretic is usually prescribed for severe CHF. Furosemide moves large volumes of fluid for excretion. It is effective even when the glomerular filtration rate (GFR) is low.
Thiazide Hydrochlorothiazide (HydroDIURIL)	Thiazide diuretics are prescribed for mild to moderate CHF. Thiazides are not effective when the GFR is low. Loop and thiazide diuretics cause potassium (K) loss; thus, potassium supplements should be given and the serum potassium levels should be closely monitored. Hypokalemia causes ventricular dysrhythmias.
Sympathomimetics *(Beta-Adrenergic Agonists)* Dopamine Dobutamine	Beta adrenergics stimulate the beta cells in the heart, increasing myocardial contractility and cardiac output. Dopamine and dobutamine have a strong positive inotropic effect (increase contractility) and can decrease afterload. These agents dilate renal blood vessels; thus, urine output is increased. However, high doses of dopamine can stimulate the alpha$_1$ adrenergic receptors, which can cause an increase in vascular resistance and an increase in afterload, which decreases cardiac output. Dobutamine does not activate the alpha$_1$ receptors. Both agents are used for short-term treatment of acute CHF.

continues on the following page

Table 19-4

(Continued)

Drug	Rationale
Phosphodiesterase Inhibitors Amrinone lactate (Inocor) Milrinone (Primacor)	These agents exert a positive inotropic effect on the heart. They increase myocardial contractility and promote vasodilation, thus decreasing afterload. They are used primarily for short-term (<24 hours) drug therapy for severe CHF.
Angiotensin-Converting Enzyme (ACE) Inhibitors Captopril (Capoten) Enalapril (Vasotec)	ACE inhibitors promote vasodilation by inhibiting angiotensin II, a potent vasoconstrictor that stimulates the release of aldosterone, causing sodium and water retention. By blocking angiotensin II, cardiac output, stroke volume, and renal blood flow are increased. Adverse effects include hypotension, hyperkalemia due to a decrease in aldosterone, and a cough of unknown origin. ACE inhibitors should not be used with potassium supplements.
Vasodilators Nitroglycerin Sodium nitroprusside Prazosin HCL (Minipress)	Vasodilators are helpful for short-term treatment of CHF. Nitrates such as nitroglycerin affect the veins, thus decreasing pooling of blood and pulmonary congestion. With nitrates, hypotension and reflex tachycardia may result. Sodium nitroprusside and prazosin can cause venous and arterial dilation. These agents decrease both preload and afterload. With use of vasodilators, the blood pressure needs to be monitored closely.

5. Monitor vital signs and ECG for changes during clinical management. Note if the client is having difficulty breathing.
6. For clients having difficulty breathing, elevate the head of the bed. This position lowers the diaphragm and increases the air space.
7. The client with CHF should not use table salt unless otherwise indicated.

❱ CLIENT MANAGEMENT FOR CHF

Assessment

- Obtain baseline vital signs and ECG to determine abnormal changes and for comparison with future vital signs and ECG readings. ·

- Assess for signs and symptoms of left-sided heart failure (overhydration or pulmonary edema), i.e., constant irritated cough, dyspnea, neck and/or hand vein engorgement, chest rales.

- Assess for signs and symptoms of right-sided heart failure, i.e., pitting peripheral edema, liver enlargement, fullness of abdomen.

- Check serum electrolyte levels, especially potassium and sodium. Use baseline electrolyte results for comparison with future serum electrolytes.

Diagnoses

- Fluid volume excess, related to cardiac decompensation secondary to left-sided and right-sided heart failure.

- Ineffective breathing patterns, related to fluid in the lung tissues.

- Impaired tissue integrity, related to fluid accumulation in the extremities and buttocks.

- Altered tissue perfusion, related to cardiopulmonary insufficiency.

Interventions

- Auscultate lung areas to detect abnormal breath sounds, such as moist rales due to lung congestion (pulmonary edema).

- Monitor vein engorgement by checking hand veins for fluid overload. Lower the hand below the heart level until the hand veins are engorged, then raise the hand above the heart level. If the hand veins remain engorged above the heart level after 15 seconds, fluid volume excess is most likely present.

- Check the feet and ankles daily in the early morning before the client rises. If edema is present, the reason is probably due to cardiac and/or renal dysfunction.

- Instruct the client not to use table salt to season foods. Salt contains sodium, which can cause water retention. Suggest other ways to enhance flavor of foods.

- Instruct the client to eat foods rich in potassium (fruits, vegetables) if the client is taking a potassium-wasting diuretic and digoxin. Hypokalemia enhances the action of digoxin and can cause digitalis toxicity (slow, irregular pulse, anorexia, nausea, vomiting).

- Assess for signs and symptoms of hypokalemia.

- Monitor breathing patterns. Note the presence of dyspnea, shortness of breath, rapid breathing, and wheezing.

- Elevate the head of the bed 30° to 75° to lower the diaphragm and increase alveoli spaces for gas exchange.

- Encourage the client to change positions frequently. Edematous tissue can break down due to hypoxia and constant pressure on skin surface.

- Provide skin care, especially to edematous areas, at least twice daily.

Evaluation/Outcome

- Evaluate the therapeutic effect of interventions to correct the underlying cause of CHF.

- Remain free of signs and symptoms of left-sided heart failure and right-sided heart failure.

- Evaluate the effectiveness of medications in reducing pulmonary and/or peripheral edema, and cardiac symptoms.

- Evaluate the dietary intake, and fluid intake and output.

- Evaluate that a support system is available for the client.

▶ DIABETES MELLITUS (DM) AND DIABETIC KETOACIDOSIS (DKA)

Diabetes mellitus results from a malfunction of the beta cells of the pancreas. The body is unable to utilize sugar due to a lack of insulin secretion from the beta cells. Approximately 11 million people in the United States are affected by some form of diabetes mellitus. There are two common types of DM: insulin-dependent diabetes mellitus (IDDM), Type I, and non-insulin-dependent diabetes mellitus (NIDDM), Type II. With NIDDM, some insulin secretion usually occurs and oral hypoglycemic agents are prescribed. Approximately 80% of this group are obese. The old term for Type I is juvenile-onset diabetes, and the old term for Type II is maturity-onset diabetes. These are misleading terms because either type of diabetes can occur in the very young or very old.

Diabetic ketoacidosis (DKA) is often associated with IDDM, Type I, and results from a severe or complete deficit of insulin secretion. DKA is characterized by a blood sugar exceeding 300 mg/dL, ketosis, a blood pH <7.30, and a bicarbonate level <14 mEq/L. **Hyperglycemic hyperosmolar nonketotic (HHNK)** syndrome is characterized by a blood sugar >500 mg/dL, dehydration, and a serum osmolality >300 mOsm/kg.

Pathophysiology

A cessation or deficit of insulin secretions limits the body's utilization of glucose. With an insulin deficit, the cells are starved of important nutrients. Fat and protein catabolism (breakdown) occurs to provide the body with needed energy. Fatty acids are released from the breakdown of adipose (fat) tissue. Acids are further broken down into ketonic acids (ketones) and acetoacetate (acetone). Because the liver cannot oxidize the excess ketones, the ketone bodies accumulate in the blood. The acetone is excreted by the lungs.

Table 19-5 describes the pathophysiologic factors associated with diabetic ketoacidosis.

Etiology

Twenty to twenty-five percent of clients in diabetic ketoacidosis (DKA) did not know they had diabetes mellitus. Selected acute stressors such as trauma, infection, and major surgical interventions can trigger the occurrence of diabetes mellitus. Untreated diabetes mellitus can lead to diabetic ketoacidosis as a result of the high blood sugar levels and lack of nutrients to the cells. Ketosis due to cellular breakdown causes the blood pH and bicarbonate levels to decrease, resulting in ketoacidosis.

Hyperosmolar hyperglycemic nonketotic (HHNK) syndrome develops in middle-age or older individuals. It is usually associated with Type II diabetics. HHNK develops more slowly than DKA. The blood sugar levels and BUN are usually greater than those with DKA. Ketosis is *not* common. Stress or injury can precipitate an HHNK state. Table 19-6 indicates the causes of DKA and HHNK.

Clinical Manifestations

The most common symptoms of DKA are extreme thirst, polyuria, weakness, and fatigue. Hyperglycemia induces osmotic diuresis. Dehydration results from diuresis; the skin is dry with poor skin turgor, and the lips are parched.

Table 19-5

Pathophysiologic Changes Associated with Diabetic Ketoacidosis

Pathophysiologic Changes	Rationale
Ketosis	Failure to metabolize glucose leads to an increase in fat catabolism and ketone bodies. Ketosis occurs when there is an excess of ketone bodies (ketonic acids) in the blood. Ketosis leads to diabetic ketoacidosis. Ketones (strong acids) combine with the sodium, causing sodium depletion. Ketone bodies are excreted as ketonuria.
Increased lactic acid	Cellular breakdown due to a lack of nutrients to the cells causes the release of lactic acid from the cells.
Increased hydrogen ions	Hydrogen ions are reabsorbed from the kidney tubules back into circulation as the bicarbonate ions are excreted. An increase in hydrogen ion concentration increases the acidotic state.
Hyperosmolality	An elevated blood sugar increases the hyperosmolality of the extracellular fluid. Because of hyperosmolality, osmotic diuresis occurs, causing the kidneys to excrete bicarbonate, potassium, and phosphorus. Also, hyperosmolality leads to the withdrawal of cellular fluid and cellular dehydration occurs.
Glycosuria	An elevation of the blood sugar, >180 mg/dL, increases the glucose concentration in the glomeruli of the kidneys. When the concentration of glucose in the glomeruli exceeds the renal threshold for tubular reabsorption, glycosuria results. Increased glucose concentration acts as an osmotic diuretic, causing diuresis.
Dehydration (cellular and extracellular)	Cellular dehydration occurs due to increased glucose concentration in the blood. Extracellular fluid increases because of the cellular fluid shift and then decreases due to osmotic diuresis. With a cellular fluid shift, potassium is lost from the cells; the extracellular potassium level may be within normal range or elevated.

Potassium, sodium, magnesium, phosphorus, and bicarbonate imbalances usually result from DKA. As cells break down because of a lack of nutrients, excess potassium moves from the cells into the extracellular compartments. When the acidotic state is corrected, potassium reenters the cells and hypokalemia may result. During early fluid loss, the sodium level may be elevated because of an increase in the

Table 19-6

Causes of Diabetic Ketoacidosis and Hyperosmolar Hyperglycemic Nonketotic Syndrome

Categories	Causes
Diabetic Ketoacidosis Insulin deficiency	Undiagnosed DM, Type I Omission of prescribed insulin
Acute incidence	Infection Trauma Major surgical interventions Pancreatitis Gastroenteritis
Miscellaneous	Hyperthyroidism Steroids (glucocorticortoids) Adrenergic agonists
Hyperosmolar Hyperglycemic Nonketotic Syndrome Insulin deficiency	Undiagnosed DM, Type II
Incidences	Stress Infection Renal or cardiovascular disease
Miscellaneous	Continuous use of total parenteral nutrition (TPN) Steroids

aldosterone secretion (sodium-retaining hormone) response. However, with continuous diuresis, the serum sodium level is decreased. The hemoglobin and hematocrit elevate in response to the fluid volume deficit (hemoconcentration). Table 19-7 describes the signs and symptoms and laboratory results related to DKA.

Classic signs and symptoms of a hypoglycemic reaction (insulin shock) include nervousness; dizziness; cold, clammy skin; tachycardia; and slurred speech. These symptoms occur when the blood sugar is 50 mg/dL or lower.

Clinical Management

Treatment modalities for DKA include: (1) vigorous fluid replacement, (2) insulin replacement, and (3) electrolyte correction. Osmotic diuresis can cause a fluid volume deficit of 4 to 8 liters of body fluid. In such a case, immediate restoration of fluid loss is essential.

Table 19-7

Clinical Manifestations of DKA

Signs and Symptoms	Rationale
Extreme Thirst *Polyuria*	Elevated blood sugar and ketones increase the serum osmolality, causing thirst and osmotic diuresis.
Weakness, Fatigue	Reduced cellular metabolism results in low energy levels.
Nausea, Vomiting	Continuous vomiting causes a loss of body fluids and electrolytes. Dehydration results.
Vital Signs Temperature elevated or N	Infection causes an elevated temperature; dehydration can cause a slightly elevated temperature.
Pulse rapid	With a loss of body fluid, the heart beats faster to compensate in order to maintain circulation. Tachycardia of greater than 140 bpm denotes a severe fluid loss.
Blood pressure slightly to severely decreased	With early fluid loss from diuresis, the blood pressure decreases by 10–15 mm Hg.
Respiration rapid, vigorous breathing	Kussmaul breathing is a compensatory mechanism to decrease H_2CO_2 (acid) by blowing off CO_2.
Poor Skin Turgor; Dry, Parched Lips; Disorientation, Confusion	Dehydration frequently results in these symptoms: poor skin turgor; dry, parched lips; and confusion.
Abdominal Pain with Tenderness	Abdominal pain usually indicates severe ketoacidosis.
Laboratory Test Results Blood sugar 300–800 mg/dL	Blood sugar level is high; at times, it is not as high as HHNK. Sugar is not metabolized and utilized by the cells.
Electrolytes Potassium N, ↓, ↑	Potassium in the cells is low, but the serum potassium level may be high due to a hemoconcentration. Normal or low levels can also occur.
Sodium N, ↓, ↑	Sodium is lost because of diuresis. Serum levels can be elevated due to dehydration.
Magnesium N, ↓, ↑ Chloride N, ↓ Phosphorus low N or ↓	Magnesium and phosphorus react the same as potassium. Chloride is excreted with sodium and water.

Note: N = normal; = ↑ elevated; ↓ = decreased; bpm = beats per minute

continues on the following page

Table 19-7

(Continued)

Signs and Symptoms	Rationale
$CO_2 \downarrow$	The serum CO_2 is a bicarbonate determinant. With the loss of bicarbonate, the serum CO_2 is greatly decreased (<14 mEq/L).
Serum osmolality 300–350 mOsm/kg	Fluid loss (dehydration) increases the serum osmolality.
Hematology Hemoglobin, hematocrit $\uparrow$ WBC $\uparrow$	Because of fluid loss, hemoconcentration results, increasing the hemoglobin and hematocrit levels. Elevated white blood cells can indicate an infection.
Arterial Blood Gases (ABGs) pH $\downarrow$ $PaCO_2 \downarrow$ $HCO_3 \downarrow$	The pH is low in the acidotic state. The $PaCO_2$ may be decreased as the lungs are expelling CO_2 (compensatory mechanism). The bicarbonate is lost through diuresis with an increase in hydrogen and ketone (acid) levels.
Urine Glycosuria Ketonuria	Glucose and ketones spill into the urine.

Note: N = normal; = $\uparrow$ elevated; $\downarrow$ = decreased; bpm = beats per minute

Fluid Replacement

In the first 24 hours, 80% of the total water and salt deficit should be replaced. There is less urgency for the other electrolytes because the rate of assimilation of the intracellular electrolytes is limited during the acidotic state. Administration of potassium must be included, but *not in early treatment* (unless indicated), because an elevated serum potassium can be toxic.

For the first hour, 1 to 2 liters of crystalloid (normal saline solution [0.9% NaCl] or lactated Ringer's solution may be rapidly infused to reestablish the fluid volume balance. This may be followed by 1 liter every hour for the next 2 hours or as indicated. Rapid fluid replacement decreases the hyperglycemic state by causing hemodilution. ECF is restored directly through intravenous therapy; however, a fluid overload in the ECF space should be avoided. ICF replacement occurs over approximately 2 days.

Insulin Replacement

Ten to fifteen years ago, massive doses of insulin were administered for the treatment of DKA. Today, less insulin is used when correcting DKA. Regular or crystalline insulin is given intravenously and/or intramuscularly. An initial bolus of 20 to 50 units of regular insulin is a common practice among many physicians. A suggested standard guideline for IV insulin replacement is an insulin bolus of 0.1 to 0.4 units of insulin per kilogram of weight followed by 0.1 units of insulin per kilogram of weight per hour in IV fluids until the blood sugar level reaches 200 to 250 mg/dL. Refer to the accompanying box for an example of this guideline.

A client weighs 154 pounds or 70 kg. The order reads: Regular insulin 0.4 U/kg as a bolus, and 0.1 U/kg per hour in normal saline solution. Using the standard guideline for an insulin bolus (0.1–0.4 × Weight in kilograms):

$$0.4 \times 70 = 28$$

Followed by the standard guideline for IV administration (0.1 × Weight in kilograms):

$$0.1 \times 70 = 7$$

The patient would receive 28 units of insulin in a bolus, followed by 7 units of insulin per hour in an IV of normal saline solution. When the blood sugar level reaches 200 to 250 mg/dL, the IV solution is usually switched to 5% dextrose in water. This prevents the possible occurrence of a hypoglycemic reaction. As the acidosis state is corrected, insulin is utilized more rapidly by the body for metabolizing sugar (glucose).

The longer the acidosis persists, the more resistant the person is likely to be to insulin. If acidosis persists, more insulin administration may be required.

Electrolyte Correction

Potassium (K) replacement should start approximately 6 to 8 hours after the first dose of insulin has been administered (intravenously or intramuscularly) and as the acidotic state is being corrected. Serum potassium levels should be taken frequently. Potassium moves back into cells as the fluid imbalance and the acidotic state are corrected.

Magnesium, phosphate, and bicarbonate serum levels should be closely monitored. If the serum magnesium level is low, hypokalemia is not fully corrected until the magnesium level is corrected.

There is some controversy related to phosphate replacement when treating DKA. Phosphates are needed for neuromuscular function; thus, serum phosphorus should be monitored along with the other electrolytes.

Another controversial issue is the use of bicarbonate therapy in the treatment of DKA. Generally, replacement of fluids and insulin corrects the acidotic state. If the pH falls below 7.1, bicarbonate replacement is usually prescribed.

A summary of the clinical management of diabetic ketoacidosis is presented in Table 19-8.

● Clinical Considerations: Diabetes Mellitus (DM) and Diabetic Ketoacidosis (DKA)

1. Check for signs and symptoms of hyperglycemia and hypo-glycemia. With hyperglycemia and DKA, extreme thirst, polyuria, weakness, and fatigue usually occur. The common signs and symp-toms of hypoglycemia are cold, clammy skin; nervousness; weak-ness; dizziness; tachycardia; slurred speech; and decreased blood pressure.

2. Assess urine output. Polyuria occurs in uncontrolled diabetes mellitus and diabetic ketoacidosis. Check urine for glycosuria and ketonuria. When blood sugar is >180 mg/dL, glycosuria usually occurs.

3. Check the serum osmolality using the formula:

$$2 \times \text{Serum Na} + \frac{\text{BUN}}{3} + \frac{\text{Glucose}}{18} = \text{serum osmolality}$$

If the serum osmolality is >296 mOsm/kg, hemoconcentration or fluid loss is occurring due to polyuria.

4. Check for signs and symptoms of fluid loss, i.e., poor skin turgor; dry, parched lips; dry, warm skin; dry mucous membranes; in-creased pulse rate; and decreased blood pressure.

5. Monitor blood sugar levels. A client with diabetes mellitus should check blood sugar level daily using a glucometer or other approved testing device. Daily insulin dose(s) may need to be increased or decreased according to blood sugar levels.

6. Monitor arterial blood gases (ABGs), particularly pH and HCO_3, when diabetic ketoacidosis is suspected. Diabetic acidosis or

Table 19-8

Treatment Modalities for Diabetic Ketoacidosis

Categories	Treatment Modalities
Fluid replacement	First 24 hours: 80% water and salt deficit replacement. First hour: 1 to 2 liters of crystalloid (normal saline solution [0.9% NaCl] or lactated Ringer's). Second and third hour: 1 liter per hour as indicated. Avoid fluid overload. Blood sugar reaches 200 to 250 mg/dL; IV fluids are switched to D_5W to avoid a possible hypoglycemic reaction. ICF replacement occurs in about 2 days.
Insulin replacement	Suggested replacement: initial bolus of regular insulin: 20 to 50 units *or* 0.1 to 0.4 U/kg. Hourly in IV fluids: 0.1 U/kg until the blood sugar level reaches 200 to 250 mg/dL. If acidosis persists, insulin resistance is occurring: More insulin administration may be needed.
Electrolyte replacement	Potassium: Replacement is initiated about 6 to 8 hours after the first dose of insulin. Monitor serum K levels frequently. Magnesium, phosphate, and bicarbonate: Monitor serum levels closely. Replace as indicated. Bicarbonate replacement is usually not indicated unless the pH is <7.1. Replacement of fluids and insulin normally corrects the acidotic state.

metabolic acidosis can occur in severely uncontrolled diabetes mellitus, Type I. A decrease in arterial pH and HCO_3 determines the severity of the acidotic state.

7. When correcting DKA, large volumes of intravenous fluids are administered. Check that a fluid overload or hypervolemia is not occurring. Signs and symptoms of hypervolemia include constant irritated cough, dyspnea, chest rales, and vein engorgement.

▶ CLIENT MANAGEMENT FOR DKA

Assessment

- Obtain the client's history of diabetes mellitus.
- Check for abnormal vital signs such as tachycardia, slightly decreased blood pressure, deep rapid breathing (Kussmaul respirations), and slightly elevated or high temperature. These can indicate dehydration and a possible acidotic state.
- Check urine for glycosuria and ketonuria. These are additional indicators of DKA.
- Assess urine output. Polyuria is an indicator of hyperglycemia and osmotic diuresis.

Diagnoses

- Fluid volume deficit, related to hyperglycemia and osmotic diuresis (polyuria).
- Altered nutrition, less than body requirements, related to insufficient utilization of glucose and nutrients.
- Altered tissue perfusion, renal, cardiopulmonary, and peripheral, related to fluid volume deficit and lack of glucose utilization.
- Fluid volume excess, related to excess administration of intravenous fluids.
- Risk for injury, cells and tissues, related to glucose intolerance and infection secondary to DKA.

Interventions

- Monitor vital signs. Changes can be indicative of fluid loss or dehydration and acidosis (rapid, thready pulse rate; slightly decreased systolic blood pressure; rapid and deep breathing (Kussmaul respiration); and a slightly elevated temperature.
- Check for other signs and symptoms of fluid loss such as poor skin turgor; dry, parched lips; dry, warm skin; and dry mucous membranes.
- Check the serum osmolality. Serum osmolality >296 mOsm/kg can indicate hemoconcentration due to fluid loss.
- Monitor blood sugar level. Levels greater than 200 mg/dL indicate hyperglycemia. Increased blood sugar levels can cause osmotic diuresis.

- Observe for signs and symptoms of hypokalemia and hyperkalemia (see Chapter 5).

- Instruct the client to monitor her blood sugar level and/or urine to denote glycosuria. For testing blood sugars, the use of a glucometer or some other approved testing device is suggested.

- Administer normal saline solution and/or a Ringer's solution as prescribed to reestablish ECF.

- Administer regular insulin intravenously as prescribed in a bolus and in IV fluids to correct insulin deficiency (see suggested guidelines in Table 19-8, page 253).

- Observe for signs and symptoms of a hypoglycemic reaction (insulin reaction or shock) from possible overcorrection of hyperglycemia. The symptoms include cold, clammy skin; nervousness; weakness; dizziness; tachycardia; low blood pressure; and slurred speech.

- Monitor urine output, heart rate, blood pressure, and chest sounds for abnormalities. Fluid deficit limits tissue perfusion and decreases circulatory volume and nutrients available to the vital organs.

- Monitor arterial blood gases (ABGs), particularly the pH, $PaCO_2$, and HCO_3. A decrease in arterial pH and HCO_3 determines the severity of the acidotic state.

Evaluation/Outcome

- Evaluate the therapeutic effect of interventions in correcting diabetic ketoacidosis. Serum osmolality, serum electrolytes, and the arterial blood gases are within normal ranges.

- The client remains free of signs and symptoms related to diabetic ketoacidosis.

- Evaluate the effectiveness of fluid, insulin, and electrolyte replacements.

- Determine that the urine output has returned to normal daily range.

▶ CHRONIC OBSTRUCTIVE PULMONARY DISEASE (COPD)

Chronic obstructive pulmonary disease (COPD), also known as chronic obstructive lung disease (COLD), is a chronic lung disease associated with airway obstruction. The narrowing of the bronchioles increases the resistance to air flow. It is the second most common cause of hospital admissions. This chronic condition can result in disabilities. Examples of COPD include emphysema, chronic bronchitis, bronchiectasis, and asthma. Smoking is the leading cause of emphysema and chronic bronchitis. Emphysema and chronic bronchitis are the common causes of COPD, and generally these disease entities coexist. Other causes of COPD include alpha-$_1$ antitrypsin deficiency (hereditary trait), chronic bacterial infection, air pollution, and inhalation of chemical irritants.

Pathophysiology

The physiologic changes associated with most types of COPD include: (1) thickening of bronchial walls caused by submucosal edema and excess mucous secretion, (2) loss of elastic recoil of lung tissue, and (3) destruction of the alveolar septa that promote overdistention and dead air space. Airway obstruction is greatest on expiration.

With advanced COPD, respiratory acidosis occurs. Because of hypoventilation, carbon dioxide is retained. Water combines with CO_2 to produce carbonic acid and a decrease in pH, resulting in respiratory acidosis. With inadequate gas exchange, CO_2 retention or hypercapnia is increased. Reduced oxygen in the blood is frequently caused by airway obstruction and alveolar hypoventilation. The thickened alveolar capillary membrane reduces oxygen diffusion. Table 19-9 lists the pathophysiologic changes and rationale associated with COPD conditions.

Etiology

Smoking, chronic or frequent acute respiratory infections, living in a densely air-polluted environment, prolonged exposure to chemical irritants, and toxic fumes are common causes of COPD. A deficiency of the protein alpha$_1$ antitrypsin, which inhibits specific proteolytic enzymes in the lung, can cause COPD. The lack of this protein is a hereditary trait; it is not the result of smoking. Table 19-10 lists the hereditary and environmental causes of COPD.

Clinical Manifestations

Early signs and symptoms of bronchitis and/or emphysema are fatigue and dyspnea on exertion. Changes in vital signs may include an increased blood pressure, increased pulse rate, and labored respirations. The expiratory phase of respiration is prolonged.

A common characteristic of COPD is a barrel-shaped chest. This is because of a loss of lung elasticity and chest wall expansion with chest

Table 19-9

Pathophysiologic Changes in Chronic Obstructive Pulmonary Disease (COPD)

Pathophysiologic Changes	Rationale
Decreased elasticity of bronchiolar walls (loss of elastic recoil)	Loss of elastic recoil causes a premature collapse of airways with expiration. Alveoli become overdistended when air is trapped in the affected lung tissue and dead air space is increased. Overdistention leads to rupture and coalescence of several alveoli.
Alveolar damage	Chronic air trapping and airway inflammation lead to weakened bronchiolar walls and alveolar disruption. Coalescence of adjacent alveoli results in bullae (parenchymal air-filled spaces >1 cm in diameter). The total area of gas exchange is greatly reduced and pulmonary hypertension may develop.
Mucous gland hyperplasia and increased mucous production	Oversecretion of mucous is commonly found in bronchitis and advanced emphysema. Increased mucous production can cause mucous plugs which lead to airway obstruction.
Inflammation of bronchial mucosa	Inflammatory infiltration and edema of the bronchial mucosa commonly occur in bronchitis, but are also found in advanced emphysema. Edema and infiltration cause thickening of bronchiolar walls.
Airway obstruction	This condition is caused primarily by narrowed bronchioles, edema, and mucous plugs. Obstruction is greatest on expiration. During inspiration bronchial lumina widen to admit air; the lumina collapse during expiration.
CO_2 retention Increased $PaCO_2 > 45$ mm Hg (hypercapnia) Norms: 35–45 mm Hg	Accumulation of carbon dioxide (CO_2) concentration in the arterial blood from inadequate gas exchange is the result of hypoventilation. CO_2 excess, >60 mm Hg, can lead to ventricular fibrillation.
Respiratory acidosis	CO_2 retention results from hypoventilation. Water combines with CO_2 to produce carbonic acid, and with increased CO_2 retention respiratory acidosis occurs [$(H_2O) + CO_2 = H_2CO_3$]. The arterial blood gases reflect pH <7.35; $PaCO_2 > 45$ mm Hg.
Hypoxemia	Hypoxemia, or reduced oxygen (O_2) in the blood, is frequently caused by airway obstruction and alveolar hypoventilation. The thickened alveolar capillary membrane reduces O_2 diffusion.
Cor pulmonale (right-sided heart failure due to pulmonary hypertension)	Destruction of alveolar tissue leads to a reduction of the size of the pulmonary capillary bed. Pulmonary hypertension occurs when $\frac{2}{3}$ to $\frac{3}{4}$ of the vascular bed is destroyed. The workload of the right ventricle is then increased, thus causing right ventricular hypertrophy and eventually CHF.
Increased red blood cell (RBC) count	Secondary polycythemia occurs as a compensatory mechanism with prolonged hypoxemia. Hemoglobin and hematocrit are increased to enhance O_2 transport.
Alpha$_1$-antitrypsin deficiency	A genetic predisposition to alpha$_1$-antitrypsin deficiency is present. An antitrypsin or trypsin inhibitor is produced in the liver. A deficit of antitrypsin allows proteolytic enzymes (released in the lungs from bacteria or phagocytic cells) to damage lung tissue. The result is emphysema.

Table 19-10

Causes of COPD

Conditions	Causes
Environmental	Smoking
	Chronic respiratory infections
	Frequent acute respiratory infections
	Living in densely air-polluted environment
	Prolonged exposure to chemical irritants
	Toxic fumes
Hereditary	Deficiency of alpha$_1$ antitrypsin protein

rigidity or dorsal kyphosis from a bent position and using accessory respiratory muscles. Respiratory infection is a complication of COPD. Bacteria grow in retained mucous secretions.

The major acid-base imbalance associated with COPD is respiratory acidosis. Arterial blood gas changes that indicate respiratory acidosis include: pH <7.35, $PaCO_2$ >45 mm Hg. Table 19-11 lists the signs and symptoms of early to advanced COPD.

Clinical Management

Low-flow oxygen is frequently needed to decrease hypoxemia. When a nasal O_2 cannula is used, the flow rate should be 1 to 2 liters per minute. If a high concentration of oxygen is delivered, the hypoxic respiratory drive is decreased.

Hydration is important in the management of COPD. Increased fluids aid in liquifying secretions and ease in the expectoration of mucous secretions. Increased fluid intake is contraindicated if CHF or cor pulmonale are present. Bronchodilators are useful to dilate the bronchial tubes, promote expectoration of mucous secretions, and improve ventilation.

Three types of chest physiotherapies are frequently prescribed. These include: (1) chest clapping for loosening thick, tenacious mucous secretions, (2) diaphragmatic breathing for increasing alveolar ventilation, and (3) pursed-lip breathing to prevent airway collapse. Table 19-12 (see page 261) lists the treatment modalities for COPD.

Table 19-11

Clinical Manifestations of COPD

Signs and Symptoms	Rationale
Chronic Fatigue	Fatigue, an early sign of COPD, is caused by hypoxia and the increased effort required to move air into and out of the lungs.
Dyspnea	Difficulty in breathing and shortness of breath following exertion are early signs of COPD. In advanced COPD, dyspnea occurs with little or no exertion.
Vital Signs	
BP increased	Increased blood pressure is due to increased sympathetic stimulation from stress.
Pulse rate increased	Increased pulse rate results from poor oxygenation. The body attempts to compensate for hypoxemia (decreased oxygen in the blood) by increasing the heart rate to carry more oxygen.
Respirations labored and increased	Loss of elasticity of lung tissue causes the bronchioles to collapse during normal expiration, thus prolonging the expiratory phase of respiration. Accessory respiratory muscles are used to improve alveolar ventilation and gas exchange.
Barrel-Shaped Chest (AP diameter > lateral diameter)	This is the result of loss of lung elasticity, chronic air trapping, and chest wall expansion with chest rigidity. It may also be compounded by dorsal kyphosis which results from a bent-forward position used to facilitate breathing. Shoulders are elevated and the neck appears to shorten. Accessory muscles of respiration are used for breathing.
Cough (productive)	A cough is usually associated with bronchitis because of the excessive secretion of the mucous glands. In emphysema a cough is associated with respiratory infection or cardiac failure. Bacterial growth in retained mucous secretions leads to repeated infections and a chronic cough.
Cyanosis	In advanced COPD, marked cyanosis is due to poor tissue perfusion, which results from hypoxemia. Signs of cyanosis may also appear when the hemoglobin is below 5 g.
Clubbing of Nails	Clubbing of nails is commonly seen in association with hypoxemia and polycythemia. It may be due to capillary dilation in an attempt to draw more oxygen to the fingertips.

continues on the following page

Table 19-11

(Continued)

Signs and Symptoms	Rationale
Laboratory Results Arterial blood gases (ABGs) pH < 7.35 $PaCO_2$ > 45 mm Hg HCO_3 > 28 mEq/L PaO_2 < 70 mm Hg BE >+ 2 (respiratory acidosis with metabolic compensation)	Increased CO_2 retention and water cause an excessive amount of carbonic acid. As a result of too much carbonic acid in the blood, acidosis develops and the pH is decreased. The $PaCO_2$ is the respiratory component of the ABGs. A decreased pH and an increased $PaCO_2$ indicate respiratory acidosis. The PaO_2 may be normal or greatly reduced, depending on the degree of distortion of ventilation/perfusion ratio. An increased bicarbonate (HCO_3) level indicates metabolic compensation to neutralize or decrease the acidotic state. A normal HCO_3 (24–28 mEq/L) indicates no compensation.
Hemoglobin (Hgb) and Hematocrit (Hct) Increased (hemoglobin may increase to 20 g)	Increased Hgb and Hct are due to hypoxemia. More hemoglobin can carry more oxygen. An elevated hemoglobin is a sign that cyanosis is more likely.
Electrolytes: Potassium, low to low normal Sodium, normal to slightly elevated	The serum potassium level may be 3.0–3.7 mEq/L and can be the result of poor dietary intake related to breathlessness, potassium-wasting diuretics, or chronic use of steroids (e.g., cortisone). Usually the sodium level is normal, but it can be elevated due to cardiac failure, excess IV saline infusions, or chronic use of steroids.

● Clinical Considerations: Chronic Obstructive Pulmonary Disease (COPD)

1. Recognize signs and symptoms of COPD, such as dyspnea, prolonged expiration, wheezing, diminished breath sounds, barrel-shaped chest, cough, and chronic fatigue.

2. Monitor arterial blood gases (ABGs). A decreased pH (<7.35) and an increased $PaCO_2$ (>45 mm Hg) are indicative of the acid-base imbalance respiratory acidosis. The compensatory (metabolic) mechanism that brings the pH close to normal value is the HCO_3.

Table 19-12

Clinical Management of COPD

Management Methods	Rationale
Oxygen (O_2)	Low-flow oxygen: 1–2 L/min with a nasal O_2 cannula or ventimask with 24 or 28% is suggested. Mechanical ventilators may be needed to decrease CO_2 retention and to aid in ventilation. Care should be taken to avoid CO_2 narcosis; O_2 that is too high decreases the hypoxic respiratory drive.
Hydration	Fluid intake should be increased to 3–4 L/day to liquify secretions and ease in expectoration *unless* cor pulmonale and/or CHF is present.
Bronchodilators: Isoproterenol (Isuprel) Metaproterenol (Alupent) Terbutaline (Brethine) Aminophylline Theophylline products	The purpose of these agents is to dilate bronchial tubes (bronchioles), expectorate mucus, and improve ventilation. Following use of a bronchodilator the client should deep breathe and cough. Bronchodilators can be administered through nebulizers (pressurized aerosols or IPPB with low-flow O_2 or compressed air), intravenously in IV fluids (aminophylline), or orally (theophylline products). Side effects of these drugs are tachycardia, cardiac dysrhythmias, and nausea/vomiting.
Antibiotics	When a respiratory infection is present, antibiotics are usually given intravenously (diluted in 50–100 mL of solution) or orally.
Chest Physiotherapy	Chest clapping loosens the thick, tenacious mucous secretions that must be "coughed up." Deep breathing and coughing should follow. Diaphragmatic breathing improves tidal volume and increases alveolar ventilation. Pursed-lip breathing prevents airway collapse so that trapped air in the alveoli can be expelled.
Exercise	Walking and stationary bicycling improve respiratory status and state of well-being.
Relaxation Techniques	Practicing relaxation techniques decreases anxiety, fear, and panic. Decreased dyspnea can result from relaxation.

3. Chest physiotherapy is helpful to mobilize secretions and improve ventilation. Types of chest physiotherapy include: chest clapping (loosens thick, tenacious mucous secretions), diaphragmatic breathing (increases alveolar ventilation), and pursed-lip breathing (prevents airway collapse).

4. Overuse of pressurized bronchodilator aerosols can cause a rebound effect.
5. COPD clients should avoid people with respiratory infections, air pollution, excess dust, pollen, and extreme hot or cold weather, all of which could cause breathlessness.
6. Hydration is important to liquify tenacious mucous secretions. Small feedings for COPD clients help prevent breathlessness that could occur when consuming large feedings.
7. Low-flow oxygen (1 to 2 liters per minute with a nasal O_2 cannula or ventimask with 24 or 28%) is suggested. Oxygen administration that is too high can decrease the hypoxic respiratory drive. Mechanical ventilators may be needed to decrease CO_2 retention and aid in ventilation.

◗ CLIENT MANAGEMENT OF COPD

Assessment

- Obtain a client history of respiratory-related problems such as dyspnea at rest and on exertion, increasing shortness of breath, wheezing, fatigue, and activity intolerance.
- Auscultate and percuss the lung areas, noting diminished breath sounds, decreased lung expansion, wheezing, crackles, and hyperresonance (hollow sound).
- Check vital signs for baseline reading to compare with future vital sign readings.
- Check the arterial blood gas (ABG) report. Compare results with the norms: pH 7.35 to 7.45, $PaCO_2$ 35 to 45 mm Hg, HCO_3 24 to 28 mEq/L, BE -2 to $+2$.

Diagnoses

- Impaired gas exchange, related to alveoli damage and the collapse of the bronchial tubes, particularly the bronchioles.
- Ineffective airway clearance, related to excess mucous secretions and the collapse of the bronchial tubes secondary to COPD.
- Ineffective breathing patterns, related to CO_2 retention and poor gas exchange secondary to COPD.
- Altered tissue perfusion, related to hypoxemia.

- Decreased cardiac output, related to breathlessness and hypoxemia secondary to COPD.

- Altered nutrition, less than body requirements, related to breathlessness.

- Anxiety related to breathlessness, dependence on others, and the treatment regime.

- Activity intolerance, related to breathlessness and fatigue.

- Self-care deficit, related to the inability to take part in ADL because of dyspnea or breathlessness.

Interventions

- Monitor ABG. A marked decrease in pH and a marked increase in $PaCO_2$ indicates respiratory acidosis.

- Monitor vital signs. Report increase in pulse rate and changes in the rate of respiration. Labored breathing is a common sign of a respiratory problem.

- Check the electrolytes and hematology findings. Elevated hemoglobin and hematocrit indicate hypoxemia.

- Monitor breath sounds and lung expansion by auscultating and percussing lung fields.

- Assist with the use of aerosol bronchodilators. Check breath sounds after use of aerosol treatments. Overuse of pressurized bronchodilator aerosol can cause a rebound effect.

- Check breath sounds for rhonchi and rales. Provide chest physiotherapy (chest clapping) for rhonchi and have client deep breathe and cough to clear bronchial secretions.

- Instruct the client on how to do breathing exercises, e.g., pursed-lip breathing to prevent airway collapse, and diaphragmatic breathing to increase alveolar ventilation.

- Monitor fluid and food intake. Hydration is important to liquify tenacious mucous secretions. Frequent small feedings may be necessary.

- Instruct the client to recognize early signs of respiratory infections, e.g., color change in sputum, elevated temperature, and coughing.

- Encourage the client to limit activities that increase the body's need for oxygen.

- Encourage the client to try mild exercises in the afternoon or when breathlessness is not severe. Avoid exercise in early mornings when mucous secretions are increased and after meals when energy is needed for digestion.
- Refer to support groups, community agencies, and/or assistance programs.

Evaluation/Outcome

- Evaluate the therapeutic effects of interventions (breathing, exercises, chest clapping, rest, bronchodilators) to correct or control COPD.
- Client remains free of signs and symptoms related to COPD.
- Evaluate effectiveness of fluid intake to aid in liquifying secretions.
- Evaluate that the laboratory findings indicative of COPD have improved.

Appendix A

Clinical Pathways

Christiana Care
Visiting Nurse Association

Page 1 of 5
Newborn Hyperbilirubinemia
Home Care Pathway

Client Name: _____
Admission #: _____
ID #: _____

Outcomes: 1. Newborn's weight stabilizes and begins to rise.
2. Bilirubin level decreases.
3. Newborn has normal skin reactions to phototherapy.

KEY	
✔ = Done ∅ = None NA = Not Applicable I = Instructed R = Reinstructed V = Variance A= Achieved	
Admission	**Discharge**
1. OASIS	Outcomes Met: 1. Y___ N___ V___ 2. Y___ N___ V___ 3. Y___ N___ V___
2. Client / Family Data	
3. HCFA Certification	Discharged to : Family _____ Other____ ED_____
4. Consent to Treat	Rehospitalized ___ Reason: _____
5. Client payment responsibilities	Plans for discharge (include MD follow - up): _____
6. Medication List	
7. DME used & company name:	
8. Bilirubin level on hospital discharge (or most recent level):____	
9. DAT=	
10. Additional Comments:	
	Physician notified of discharge:_____
	Spoke to:_____ Date/Time:_____
	Nurse's Signature:_____ Date:_____

Assessment Visit # 1 Date:

1. Vital signs: Temperature_____
   Apical pulse_____
   Regular_____
   Irregular_____
   Murmur_____ (S1/S2?)
   Respirations_____

2. STATE: Deep Sleep____ Light Sleep____ Drowsy____
   Alert, Eyes Bright____ Eyes Open, Motor Activity ____
   Crying (consolable)____ Crying (not consolable)____

3. Presence of NB reflexes: Moro____ TN____
   Root____ Suck____
   Grasp____ Plantar____

4. Fontanels:
   Flat_____ Depressed_____ Bulging_____

5. Skin color, including which areas of the skin area jaundiced:

   Skin turgor:_____

   Areas of pressure/ skin breakdown:_____

   Signs of birth trauma (describe and measure):_____

6. Current weight (Calibrate scale using known weight measure prior to weighing newborn):
   _____ weight loss over_____ (hours, days)
   _____ weight gain over_____ (hours, days)

Nurse's Signature:
Print Name: **Initial:**

Assessment Visit # 2 Date:

1. Vital signs: Temperature_____
   Apical pulse_____
   Regular_____
   Irregular_____
   Murmur_____ (S1/S2?)
   Respirations_____

2. STATE: Deep Sleep____ Light Sleep____ Drowsy____
   Alert, Eyes Bright____ Eyes Open, Motor Activity ____
   Crying (consolable)____ Crying (not consolable)____

3. Presence of NB reflexes: Moro____ TN____
   Root____ Suck____
   Grasp____ Plantar____

4. Fontanels:
   Flat_____ Depressed_____ Bulging_____

5. Skin color, including which areas of the skin area jaundiced:

   Skin turgor:_____

   Areas of pressure/ skin breakdown:_____

   Signs of birth trauma (describe and measure):_____

6. Current weight (Calibrate scale using known weight measure prior to weighing newborn):
   _____ weight loss over_____ (hours, days)
   _____ weight gain over_____ (hours, days)

Nurse's Signature:
Print Name: **Initial:**

Courtesy of Christiana Care Visiting Nurse Association, New Castle, DE

Christiana Care
Visiting Nurse Association

Page 2 of 5
Newborn Hyperbilirubinemia
Home Care Pathway

Client Name:_____
ID #:_____

Assessment Visit # 1 Date:	Assessment Vist #2 Date:
7. Feeding Breastfeeding:_____minutes, q._____hour(s) Do breast(s) feel lighter after feeding? Yes___No__ Is suck strong and coordinated? Yes___No___ Formula Type:_____ Amount and frequency:_____	7. Feeding Breastfeeding:_____minutes, q._____hour(s) Do breast(s) feel lighter after feeding? Yes___No__ Is suck strong and coordinated? Yes___No___ Formula Type:_____ Amount and frequency:_____
8. Elimination Diapers wet:____(over_____hours) Soiled:____(over_____hours)	8. Elimination Diapers wet:____(over_____hours) Soiled:____(over_____hours)
9. Circumcision? Yes_____No____N/A____	9. Circumcision? Yes_____No____N/A____
Goals: ☐ Newborn is normothermic. ☐ Adequate # wet/soiled diapers (If BF: 2 wet, 2 soiled on day 2). ☐ Vital signs wnl. ☐ Newborn is alert and responsive. ☐ Skin is intact. ☐ No S/Sx of dehydration. ☐ Newborn is feeding well. Comments:_____	**Goals:** ☐ Newborn is normothermic. ☐ Adequate # wet/soiled diapers (If BF: 2 wet, 2 soiled on day 2). ☐ Vital signs wnl. ☐ Newborn is alert and responsive. ☐ Skin is intact. ☐ No S/Sx of dehydration. ☐ Newborn is feeding well. Comments:_____
Treatment Visit	**Treatment Visit**

1. Heelstick for serum bilirubin level=_____
   Area: L heel____R heel____
   Medial____Lateral____
2. Laboratory should call physician with results.
3. Home care nurse should communicate with physician for further orders (Record communication with MD office here: Name of person spoken to, date/time):_____
4. Phototherapy unit placed in accordance with manufacturer's guidelines. Intensity selected is HIGH.
   Single_____ or Double_____Phototherapy
Goals:
 ☐ Bilirubin level is decreasing.
 ☐ Skin is intact at heelstick site(s).
 ☐ Phototherapy unit is correctly placed.
 	
Comments:_____
	1. Heelstick for serum bilirubin level=_____
	   Area: L heel____R heel____
	   Medial____Lateral____
	2. Laboratory should call physician with results.
	3. Home care nurse should communicate with physician for further orders (Record communication with MD office here: Name of person spoken to, date/time):_____
	4. Phototherapy unit placed in accordance with manufacturer's guidelines. Intensity selected is HIGH.
	   Single_____ or Double_____Phototherapy
	Goals:
	 ☐ Bilirubin level is decreasing.
	 ☐ Skin is intact at heelstick site(s).
	 ☐ Phototherapy unit is correctly placed.
	
	Comments:_____

Medications	**Medications**
Record on Medication List. Untoward side effects of medications:_____	Document changes on Medication List. Untoward side effects of medications:_____
Goal: ☐ Medications given by caregiver as directed.	**Goal:** ☐ Medications given by caregiver as directed.
Nurse's Signature:	**Nurse's Signature:**
Print Name: **Initial:**	**Print Name:** **Initial:**

Courtesy of Christiana Care Visiting Nurse Association, New Castle, DE

Christiana Care
Visiting Nurse Association

Newborn Hyperbilirubinemia
Home Care Pathway

Client Name:_____
ID#:_____

Instruction Visit 1 Date:	Instruction Visit 2 Date:

1. Instruct caregiver in the following:
• Cause of newborn hyperbilirubinemia
• Normal breakdown mechanism of hemoglobin and excretion (urobilinogen in urine: dark urine; stercobilinogen in stool: brown stool)
• Record-keeping: Axillary temperature
    Oral intake
    Elimination
	1. Instruct caregiver in the following:
	• Cause of newborn hyperbilirubinemia
	• Normal breakdown mechanism of hemoglobin and excretion (urobilinogen in urine: dark urine; stercobilinogen in stool: brown stool)
	• Record-keeping: Axillary temperature
	    Oral intake
	    Elimination

2. Instruct on use of phototherapy unit(s): • Keep newborn on phototherapy 23 out of 24 hours • Phototherapy unit should be on highest intensity • Changing light bulb • Unit should be placed so ventilation is not obstructed	2. Instruct on use of phototherapy unit(s): • Keep newborn on phototherapy 23 out of 24 hours • Phototherapy unit should be on highest intensity • Changing light bulb • Unit should be placed so ventilation is not obstructed
3. Instruct caregiver on skin care: • Avoidance of skin lotion • Appearance of maculopapular rash is common and disappears spontaneously • Reporting extreme skin erythema, dryness, and blistering	3. Instruct caregiver on skin care: • Avoidance of skin lotion • Appearance of maculopapular rash is common and disappears spontaneously • Reporting extreme skin erythema, dryness, and blistering
4. Instruct caregiver to do the following: • Check axillary temperature qid • Report 97.4 <T>99.4F to VNA nurse • Offer frequent feedings • If breastfeeding, encourage at least 8 feedings daily • Positioning • Report decreased intake or urine output or projectile vomiting to VNA nurse	4. Instruct caregiver to do the following: • Check axillary temperature qid • Report 97.4 <T>99.4F to VNA nurse • Offer frequent feedings • If breastfeeding, encourage at least 8 feedings daily • Positioning • Report decreased intake or urine output or projectile vomiting to VNA nurse
Patient education materials provided/used:_____	Patient education materials provided/used:_____
Goals: ❑ **Newborn is properly placed on phototherapy unit(s).** ❑ **Caregiver demonstrates ability to assemble and use phototherapy unit(s).** ❑ **Caregiver verbalizes knowledge of disease, purpose, and phototherapy procedure.** Comments:_____	**Goals:** ❑ **Newborn is properly placed on phototherapy unit(s).** ❑ **Caregiver demonstrates ability to assemble and use phototherapy unit(s).** ❑ **Caregiver verbalizes knowledge of disease, purpose, and phototherapy procedure.** Comments:_____
Nurse's Signature:	**Nurse's Signature:**
Print Name: **Initial**	**Print Name:** **Initial:**

Courtesy of Christiana Care Visiting Nurse Association, New Castle, DE

**Christiana Care
Visiting Nurse Association**

Page 4 of 5
Newborn Hyperbilirubinemia
Home Care Pathway

Client Name:_____
ID#:_____

Psychosocial Visit 1 Date:	Psychosocial Visit 2 Date:
1. Comprehension (Ability to grasp concepts and respond to?) Exhibits: High____ Medium____ Low____ 2. Motivation Level (Code: F=Family/Caregiver C=Client) ____Asks questions ____Eager to learn ____Extremely anxious ____Uncooperative ____Seems uninterested ____Denies educational need 3. Language barrier:____Yes____No 4. Literate:____Yes____No Comments:_____	1. Family Relationships: _____ _____ _____ _____ _____ 2. Family Stressors: _____ _____ 3. Financial Problems: _____
Goal: ❑ Caregiver is comfortable using phototherapy unit(s) **Referrals / Interdisciplinary Services** 1. Smoking cessation for caregiver/ family 2. MSW 3. Lactation Consultant 4. La Leche League International: 1(800)La Leche (525-3243) 5. Nursing Mother's, Inc.: (302)733-0973 6. The Warm Line: (302)762-8938 7. Other:_____ **Goal:** ❑ Client / Family can list resources available. Comments:_____	4. Other: _____ **Goal:** ❑ Caregiver / Family gaining increasing sense of control over treatment of hyperbilirubinemia. **Referrals / Interdisciplinary Services** 1. Smoking cessation for caregiver/ family 2. MSW 3. Lactation Consultant 4. La Leche League International: 1(800)La Leche (525-3243) 5. Nursing Mother's, Inc.: (302)733-0973 6. The Warm Line: (302)762-8938 7. Other:_____ **Goal:** ❑ Client / Family can list resources available. Comments:_____
Nurse's Signature_____	**Nurses's Signature:**_____
Print Name:_____ **Initial:**	**Print Name:**_____ **Initial:**

Courtesy of Christiana Care Visiting Nurse Association, New Castle, DE

Christiana Care
Visiting Nurse Association

Page 5 of 5
Clinical Pathway for Home Care: Hyperbilirubinemia
Outcome Record

Client Name:_____
Admission #:_____
ID #:_____

ICD9 Code:_____
Pathway Start Date:_____ Pathway Stop Date:_____   # of Home Visits:_____

Client Variance
❑ A1 Readmitted to hospital ❑ A5 Other_____   ❑ A2 Death   ❑ A3 Caregiver noncompliance   ❑ A4 Continues home care r/t_____

System Variance Internal	❑ B1 Equipment not available ❑ B2 Visit delay impending progress or treatment
System Variance External	❑ B3 Insurance problem ❑ B4 Transportation problem

Nurse's Initials	Date	Visit Day	Variance Code	Variance/Explanation/Comments	Variance Caused Delay (Y/N)	Action Taken

Note: Y= Yes, N= No

Nurse's Signature:	Initials:	Nurse's Signature:	Initials:
Print Name:		Print Name:	
Nurse's Signature:	Initials:	Nurse's Signature:	Initials:
Print Name:		Print Name:	
Nurse's Signature:	Initials:	Nurse's Signature:	Initials:
Print Name:		Print Name:	

Hyperout 698 Gale

Courtesy of Christiana Care Visiting Nurse Association, New Castle, DE

Clinical Pathway -   ┌─ **DRAFT** ─┐   CONGESTIVE HEART FAILURE

ACUTE PHASE - EMERGENCY DEPARTMENT	DATE ___/___/___

Disclaimer for Pathways and Guidelines: Clinical Pathways and Guidelines are developed by a multidisciplinary team. They are guidelines for care. They are not compulsory or mandatory plans of treatment or standards of care. When considering individual patient needs, alternative independent clinical assessments and judgements may be necessary.

BELOW: SELECT SHIFT & INITIAL

		0700-1500	1500-2300	2300-0700
Assessment	H&P per ED Protocol.	☐ _____	☐ _____	☐ _____
	Vital signs & multisystem assessment per ED protocol	☐ _____	☐ _____	☐ _____
	Advanced directives addressed	☐ _____	☐ _____	☐ _____
	Guideline I: S&S Diagnosis of CHF	☐ _____	☐ _____	☐ _____
	Guideline II: CHF Pathway/Risk Stratification.	☐ _____	☐ _____	☐ _____
	Guideline VI: Level of Care for CHF Patients	☐ _____	☐ _____	☐ _____
Treatments	Continuous cardiac monitoring	☐ _____	☐ _____	☐ _____
	Weight prior to diuresis (if appropriate)	☐ _____	☐ _____	☐ _____
	Foley catheter as indicated	☐ _____	☐ _____	☐ _____
Tests/Labs	**Guideline III / IV: Diagnostic Procedures in New Onset/Established CHF** (EKG,CXR,CBC, complete chemistry profile, Mg, thyroid function, other as indicated)	☐ _____	☐ _____	☐ _____
	Pulse Oximetry per protocol	☐ _____	☐ _____	☐ _____
Medications/IVs	IV access	☐ _____	☐ _____	☐ _____
	Oxygen therapy per protocol	☐ _____	☐ _____	☐ _____
	Guideline IX: Diuresis	☐ _____	☐ _____	☐ _____
	Evaluate patient's routine medications	☐ _____	☐ _____	☐ _____
Consults	Cardiology consult as indicated	☐ _____	☐ _____	☐ _____
Nutrition	NPO except for medications	☐ _____	☐ _____	☐ _____
Activity/Safety	Bedrest	☐ _____	☐ _____	☐ _____
	High Fowlers position	☐ _____	☐ _____	☐ _____
Discharge Planning	Responsible support person identified	☐ _____	☐ _____	☐ _____
	Residence prior to admission identified	☐ _____	☐ _____	☐ _____
Patient/Family Teaching Outcomes	Verbalizes understanding of: Treatment plan and need for admission. . .	☐ _____	☐ _____	☐ _____
	Importance of notifying the staff when experiencing SOB or chest pain	☐ _____	☐ _____	☐ _____
	Need for limited activity.	☐ _____	☐ _____	☐ _____
Clinical Processes/ Outcomes	If patient meets criteria, meds given in ED:			
	● Furosemide	☐ _____	☐ _____	☐ _____
	● Bumetanide.	☐ _____	☐ _____	☐ _____
	● Morphine.	☐ _____	☐ _____	☐ _____
	● Nitrates	☐ _____	☐ _____	☐ _____
	● Heparin	☐ _____	☐ _____	☐ _____
	Documentation of support person on record. Residence and telephone documented on record	☐ _____	☐ _____	☐ _____

INITIAL	SIGNATURE	TITLE	INITIAL	SIGNATURE	TITLE

PHYSICIAN SIGNATURE: _____

COPYRIGHT 1998 St. Francis Hospital, INC   1/98   H:\ceu\Pathways\CHF\pathway.doc

Courtesy of St. Francis Hospital, Wilmington, Delaware

Clinical Pathway -

DRAFT

CONGESTIVE HEART FAILURE

ACUTE PHASE - DAY 1   (ICU/TELEMETRY/MS UNIT)   DATE ____ / ____ / ____

(ADMISSION DAY or OBSERVATION DAY [0-24 hrs])

Disclaimer for Pathways and Guidelines: Clinical Pathways and Guidelines are developed by a multidisciplinary team. They are guidelines for care. They are not compulsory or mandatory plans of treatment or standards of care. When considering individual patient needs, alternative independent clinical assessments and judgements may be necessary.

		BELOW: SELECT SHIFT & INITIAL		
		0700-1500	1500-2300	2300-0700
Assessment	Vital signs & systems assessment per unit protocol	☐ ____	☐ ____	☐ ____
	Advanced directives addressed	☐ ____	☐ ____	☐ ____
	Monitor for signs & symptoms of SOB, JVD, rales, peripheral edema, S3,S4, murmur, arrhythmias .	☐ ____	☐ ____	☐ ____
	Guideline VI: Level of Care for CHF Patients . . .	☐ ____	☐ ____	☐ ____
Treatments	Continuous cardiac monitoring as indicated	☐ ____	☐ ____	☐ ____
	Weight q AM	☐ ____	☐ ____	☐ ____
	Intake & output	☐ ____	☐ ____	☐ ____
Tests/Labs	Pulse Oximetry per protocol	☐ ____	☐ ____	☐ ____
	Guideline III: Diagnostic Procedures in New Onset CHF.	☐ ____	☐ ____	☐ ____
	Guideline IV: Diagnostic Procedures in Established CHF.	☐ ____	☐ ____	☐ ____
	Guideline V: Assessment of LV Function in CHF	☐ ____	☐ ____	☐ ____
Medications/IVs	IV access	☐ ____	☐ ____	☐ ____
	Oxygen therapy per protocol	☐ ____	☐ ____	☐ ____
	Guideline IX: Diuresis	☐ ____	☐ ____	☐ ____
	Guideline X: ACE Inhibitors	☐ ____	☐ ____	☐ ____
	Guideline XII: Digoxin	☐ ____	☐ ____	☐ ____
	Guideline XIII: Indications for Anticoagulation .	☐ ____	☐ ____	☐ ____
	Guideline XIV, XV, XVI, and XVII.	☐ ____	☐ ____	☐ ____
	Patient's routine medications as indicated	☐ ____	☐ ____	☐ ____
Consults	Cardiology consult as indicated	☐ ____	☐ ____	☐ ____
Nutrition	Cardiac diet as tolerated (additional Na and fluid restrictions as indicated)	☐ ____	☐ ____	☐ ____
	Nutrition screen, Diet Teaching Needs Assessment	☐ ____	☐ ____	☐ ____
Activity/Safety	Bedrest with BRP/bedside commode	☐ ____	☐ ____	☐ ____
	Fall risk assessment completed	☐ ____	☐ ____	☐ ____
	Maintain semi-Fowlers position	☐ ____	☐ ____	☐ ____
Discharge Planning	Care management assessment:			
	• Evaluation of support system and discharge needs	☐ ____	☐ ____	☐ ____
	• Preadmission compliance with diet and medication evaluated	☐ ____	☐ ____	☐ ____
	• Initial discharge plan addressed, with patient and caregiver.	☐ ____	☐ ____	☐ ____
	• Need for DME and home weight scale identified.	☐ ____	☐ ____	☐ ____
Patient/Family Teaching Outcomes	• Verbalizes basic understanding of disease process (reason for SOB and decreased activity level, etc.)	☐ ____	☐ ____	☐ ____
Clinical Processes/ Outcomes	• Decreasing SOB	☐ ____	☐ ____	☐ ____
	• JVD decreasing	☐ ____	☐ ____	☐ ____
	• Improved breath sounds	☐ ____	☐ ____	☐ ____
	• Negative fluid balance >500(8hr), 750(12hr) . . .	☐ ____	☐ ____	☐ ____
	• LV Function ordered or documented in record (as appropriate).	☐ ____	☐ ____	☐ ____
	• O₂ Sat maintained > 92%	☐ ____	☐ ____	☐ ____

INITIAL	SIGNATURE		TITLE	INITIAL	SIGNATURE		TITLE

PHYSICIAN SIGNATURE: _____

COPYRIGHT 1998 St. Francis Hospital, INC   1/98   H:\ceu\Pathways\CHF\pathway.doc

Courtesy of St. Francis Hospital, Wilmington, Delaware

Clinical Pathway -

| DRAFT |

CONGESTIVE HEART FAILURE

IMPROVING PHASE - DAY 2 ICU/TELEMETRY/MS UNIT   DATE ____/____/____

Disclaimer for Pathways and Guidelines: Clinical Pathways and Guidelines are developed by a multidisciplinary team. They are guidelines for care. They are not compulsory or mandatory plans of treatment or standards of care. When considering individual patient needs, alternative independent clinical assessments and judgements may be necessary.

		BELOW: SELECT SHIFT & INITIAL		
		0700-1500	1500-2300	2300-0700
Assessment	Vital signs & multisystem assessment per unit protocol..........................	☐ _____	☐ _____	☐ _____
	Monitor for signs & symptoms of SOB, JVD, rales, peripheral edema......................	☐ _____	☐ _____	☐ _____
	Guideline VI: Level of Care for CHF Patients ...			
Treatments	Continuous cardiac monitoring as indicated	☐ _____	☐ _____	☐ _____
	Weight q AM............................	☐ _____	☐ _____	☐ _____
	Intake & output q 8 hours	☐ _____	☐ _____	☐ _____
	D/C foley if indicated	☐ _____	☐ _____	☐ _____
Tests/Labs	Guideline III: Diagnostic Procedures in New Onset CHF............................	☐ _____	☐ _____	☐ _____
	Guideline IV: Diagnostic Procedures in Established CHF.......................	☐ _____	☐ _____	☐ _____
	Guideline V: Assessment of LV Function in CHF			
	Pulse Oximetry per protocol	☐ _____	☐ _____	☐ _____
Medications/IVs	Oxygen therapy per protocol	☐ _____	☐ _____	☐ _____
	Guideline IX: Diuresis	☐ _____	☐ _____	☐ _____
	Guideline X: ACE Inhibitors	☐ _____	☐ _____	☐ _____
	Guideline XII: Digoxin	☐ _____	☐ _____	☐ _____
	Guideline XIII: Anticoagulation in CHF	☐ _____	☐ _____	☐ _____
	Guideline XIV, XV, XVI, and XVII.	☐ _____	☐ _____	☐ _____
	Patient's routine medications as indicated			
Consults	Nutrition for Level 4 Malnutrition Risk and diet teaching............................	☐ _____	☐ _____	☐ _____
Nutrition	Cardiac diet (additional Na and fluid restrictions as indicated)	☐ _____	☐ _____	☐ _____
Activity/Safety	OOB X 3 with assistance (meals in chair, remain up for 30 minutes).........................	☐ _____	☐ _____	☐ _____
	Encourage high to semi-Fowlers position when in bed and during meals	☐ _____	☐ _____	☐ _____
Discharge Planning	• Care manager reassessment of discharge plan, assess needs for Home O₂ and refer as indicated..............................	☐ _____	☐ _____	☐ _____
	• Assess need for Home Health, Telemanagement, Cardiac Rehab referral....................	☐ _____	☐ _____	☐ _____
Patient/Family Teaching Outcomes	• Demonstrates understanding of activity level....	☐ _____	☐ _____	☐ _____
	• Medication instructions initiated..............	☐ _____	☐ _____	☐ _____
	• Verbalizes understanding of relationship of increased Na and fluid intake with SOB, weight gain, and peripheral edema.................	☐ _____	☐ _____	☐ _____
	• Verbalizes rationale for daily weight monitoring..			
Clinical Processes/ Outcomes	• Decreased weight	☐ _____	☐ _____	☐ _____
	• Increased activity without increased SOB.......	☐ _____	☐ _____	☐ _____
	• Negative fluid balance.....................	☐ _____	☐ _____	☐ _____
	• ECHO completed........................	☐ _____	☐ _____	☐ _____
	• Receiving Ace inhibitors..................	☐ _____	☐ _____	☐ _____
	• Receiving digoxin.......................	☐ _____	☐ _____	☐ _____
	• Receiving diuretics......................			

INITIAL	SIGNATURE	TITLE	INITIAL	SIGNATURE	TITLE

PHYSICIAN SIGNATURE: _____

COPYRIGHT 1998 St. Francis Hospital, INC   1/98   H:\ceu\Pathways\CHF\pathway.doc

Courtesy of St. Francis Hospital, Wilmington, Delaware

Clinical Pathway -

| DRAFT |

CONGESTIVE HEART FAILURE

DISCHARGE PHASE - DAY 3, 4, ___ (TELEMETRY/MS UNIT)   DATE ___/___/___

Disclaimer for Pathways and Guidelines: Clinical Pathways and Guidelines are developed by a multidisciplinary team. They are guidelines for care. They are not compulsory or mandatory plans of treatment or standards of care. When considering individual patient needs, alternative independent clinical assessments and judgements may be necessary.

		BELOW: SELECT SHIFT & INITIAL		
		0700-1500	1500-2300	2300-0700
Assessment	Vital signs & system assessment per unit protocol	☐ _____	☐ _____	☐ _____
	Advanced directives addressed	☐ _____	☐ _____	☐ _____
	Guideline VI: Level of Care for CHF Patients	☐ _____	☐ _____	☐ _____
	Guideline VIII: NYHA Classification Circle - I , II , III, IV)	☐ _____	☐ _____	☐ _____
Treatments	Continuous cardiac monitoring as indicated . . .	☐ _____	☐ _____	☐ _____
	Weight q AM	☐ _____	☐ _____	☐ _____
	Intake and output q 8 hours	☐ _____	☐ _____	☐ _____
Tests/Labs	Pulse Oximetry per protocol	☐ _____	☐ _____	☐ _____
Medications/IVs	Oxygen Therapy per protocol	☐ _____	☐ _____	☐ _____
	Guideline IX: Diureses	☐ _____	☐ _____	☐ _____
	Guideline X: Ace Inhibitors	☐ _____	☐ _____	☐ _____
	Guideline XII: Digoxin	☐ _____	☐ _____	☐ _____
	Guideline XIII: Anticoagulation in CHF	☐ _____	☐ _____	☐ _____
	Guideline XIV, XV, XVI, and XVII.	☐ _____	☐ _____	☐ _____
	Patient's routine medications as indicated	☐ _____	☐ _____	☐ _____
Consults	High-risk patients meeting nutrition needs.	☐ _____	☐ _____	☐ _____
	Diet education completed.	☐ _____	☐ _____	☐ _____
Nutrition	Cardiac diet (additional Na and fluid restrictions as indicated)	☐ _____	☐ _____	☐ _____
Activity/Safety	OOB and ambulating as tolerated	☐ _____	☐ _____	☐ _____
	Meals in chair, remain up for 30 minutes	☐ _____	☐ _____	☐ _____
	Encourage self care	☐ _____	☐ _____	☐ _____
Discharge Planning	Discharge resources identified and referrals made as indicated:			
	• Smoking cessation program	☐ _____	☐ _____	☐ _____
	• Home Health referral.	☐ _____	☐ _____	☐ _____
	• Cardiac Rehabilitation.	☐ _____	☐ _____	☐ _____
Patient/Family Teaching Outcomes	Verbalizes understanding of:			
	• Discharge medication regimen, action, side effects, drug and food interaction.	☐ _____	☐ _____	☐ _____
	• Importance of monitoring daily wt - notify MD with increase of 3lbs in weight and/or increasing SOB.	☐ _____	☐ _____	☐ _____
	• Cardiac diet as indicated.	☐ _____	☐ _____	☐ _____
Clinical Processes/ Outcomes	Resp. rate at baseline with increased activity. . .	☐ _____	☐ _____	☐ _____
	Stable rate, rhythm, & BP with increased activity.	☐ _____	☐ _____	☐ _____
	• Receiving ACE inhibitors.	☐ _____	☐ _____	☐ _____
	• Receiving digoxin	☐ _____	☐ _____	☐ _____
	• Receiving diuretics.	☐ _____	☐ _____	☐ _____
	• **Guideline VII: Discharge Criteria met :** (Y = D/C) (N= reapply next day).	☐ _____	☐ _____	☐ _____

INITIAL	SIGNATURE	TITLE	INITIAL	SIGNATURE	TITLE

PHYSICIAN SIGNATURE: _____

COPYRIGHT 1998 St. Francis Hospital, INC   1/98   H:\ceu\Pathways\CHF\pathway.doc

Courtesy of St. Francis Hospital, Wilmington, Delaware

Appendix B

Summary of Acid-Base Imbalances

Metabolic Acidosis	Metabolic Alkalosis
Clinical Manifestations	
Kussmaul breathing (rapid and vigorous)	Shallow breathing
Flushing of the skin (capillary dilation)	Tetanylike symptoms
Decrease in heart rate and cardiac output	Irritability, confusion
Nausea, vomiting, abdominal pain	Vomiting
Dehydration	
Laboratory Findings	
Bicarbonate deficit	*Bicarbonate excess*
pH$<$7.35, HCO$_3$$<$24 mEq/L,	pH$>$7.45, HCO$_3$$>$28 mEq/L, BE$>$+2,
BE$<$$-$2, plasma CO$_2$$<$22 mEq/L	plasma CO$_2$ $>$32 mEq/L
Causes	
Diabetic acidosis, severe diarrhea or starvation, tissue trauma, renal and heart failure, shock, severe infection	Peptic ulcer, vomiting, gastric suction

Respiratory Acidosis	Respiratory Alkalosis
Clinical Manifestations	
Dyspnea, inadequate gas exchange	Rapid, shallow breathing
Flushing and warm skin	Tetanylike symptoms (numbness, tingling
Tachycardia	of fingers)
Weakness	Palpitations
	Vertigo
Laboratory Findings	
Carbonic acid excess (CO$_2$ retention)	*Carbonic acid deficit*
pH$<$7.35, PaCO$_2$ $>$45 mm Hg	pH$>$7.45, PaCO$_2$ $<$35 mm Hg
Causes	
COPD (emphysema, chronic bronchitis, severe asthma), narcotics, anesthetics, barbiturates, pneumonia, chest injuries	Anxiety, hysteria, drug toxicity, fever, pain, brain tumors, early salicylate poisoning, excessive exercise

Appendix C

Clinical Problems Associated with Fluid Imbalances

Clinical Problems	ECFVD	ECFVE	ECFV Shift	ICFVE
Gastrointestinal				
Vomiting and diarrhea	+			
GI fistula	+			
GI suctioning	+			
Increased salt intake	+			
Intestinal obstruction	+		+	
Perforated ulcer	+		+	
Excessive hypotonic fluids, oral and intravenous				+
Renal				
Renal failure		+		
Renal disease		+		
Cardiac				
Congestive heart failure		+		
Miscellaneous				
Brain tumor/injury				+
Fever	+			
Profused diaphoresis	+			
SIADH (syndrome of inappropriate antidiuretic hormone)		Initially +		+
Burns	+	+	+	
Diabetic ketoacidosis	+			
Ascites (cirrhosis)		+	+	
Venous obstruction		+		
Sprain			+	
Massive trauma	+		+	
Drugs				
Cortisone group of drugs		+		

Appendix D

Clinical Problems Associated with Electrolyte Imbalances

Clinical Problems	Potassium	Sodium	Calcium	Magnesium	Phosphorus
Gastrointestinal					
Vomiting and diarrhea	K↓	Na↓	Ca↓	Mg↓	P↓
Malnutrition	K↓	Na↓	Ca↓	Mg↓	P↓
Anorexia nervosa	K↓	Na↓	Ca↓	Mg↓	P↓
Intestinal fistula	K↓	Na↓		Mg↓	P↓
GI surgery	K↓	Na↓		Mg↓	P↓
Chronic alcoholism	K↓	Na↓	Ca↓	Mg↓	P↓
Lack of vitamin D			Ca↓		
Hyperphosphatemia			Ca↓		
Transfusion of citrated blood			Ca↓		
Cardiac					
Myocardial infarction	K↓	Na↓		Mg↓	
		Hypervolemia			
Congestive heart failure (CHF)	K↓/N	Na↑		Mg↓/N	
Endocrine					
Cushing's syndrome	K↓	Na↑		Mg↓	
Addison's disease	K↑	Na↓		Mg↑	
Diabetic ketoacidosis	K↑	Na↑/↓	Ca↓	Mg↑	P↓/N
	Diuresis K↓		(ionized)	Diuresis Mg↓	
Parathyroidism					
Hypo:			Ca↓		P↑
Hyper:			Ca↑		P↓
Renal					
Acute renal failure	Oliguria K↑	Na↑		Mg↑	P↑
	Diuresis K↓				
Chronic renal failure	K↑	Na↑	Ca↑/↓	Mg↑	P↑
Miscellaneous					
Cancer	K↓/↑	Na↓	Ca↑	Mg↓	P↓
Bone destruction			Ca↑		
Burns	K↓/↑	Na↓	Ca↓	Mg↓	P↓
Acute pancreatitis			Ca↓		
SIADH (syndrome of inappropriate antidiuretic hormone)		Na↓			
Metabolic acidosis	K↑		Ca↓		
Metabolic alkalosis	K↓				
Drugs					
Diuretics					
Potassium wasting	K↓	Na↓	Ca↑/↓	Mg↓	
Potassium sparing	K↑/N	Na↓		Mg↓	
ACE inhibitors	K↑	Na↓/N			

Appendix E

Clinical Assessment Tool: Fluid, Electrolyte, and Acid-Base Imbalances

This assessment tool can be used for assessing fluid, electrolyte, and acid-base imbalances in all clinical settings.

A. Health history of the clinical problem
  1. Chief complaint
  2. History of the present illness
     a. Date of onset
     b. Duration
     c. Effects of bodily function
     d. Treatment and medications—effective or noneffective
  3. Past history of clinical condition
B. Fluid balance assessment
  1. Skin turgor
  2. Mucous membrane
  3. Vital signs—P↑, BP↓, T sl↑
  4. Insensible fluid loss
     a. Diaphoresis
     b. Hyperventilation
  5. Body weight loss—2.2 pounds = 1 liter of water
  6. Intake and output
     a. Intake: oral; IV fluids
     b. Output: urine; stool; GI fluids; blood; wound
  7. Edema
  8. Behavioral changes—confusion and irritability (ECFV↓ and ICFV↑)
  9. Neck and/or hand vein engorgement
  10. Chest sounds—rales
  11. Laboratory results
     a. Serum osmolality   <280 mOsm/kg, overhydration
                            >295 mOsm/kg, dehydration

    b. Hemoglobin   <12 g/dL, anemia
                                              >17 g/dL, dehydration
    c. Hematocrit   >52%, possible dehydration
    d. BUN (10–25 mg/dL   >25–35 mg/dL, possible
         range)   dehydration
    e. Creatinine (0.7–   >1.5 mg/dL, possible
         1.4 mg/dL range)   dehydration; > 1.7 possible renal insufficiency

C. Electrolyte balance assessment
  1. Serum electrolytes
    a. Potassium: 3.5–5.3 mEq/L
    b. Sodium: 135–146 mEq/L
    c. Calcium: 4.5–5.5 mEq/L; 9–11 mg/dL; 2.3–2.8 mmol/L (SI units)
       Ionized calcium: 2.2–2.5 mEq/L; 4.4–5.0 mg/dL; 1.1–1.24 mmol/L
    d. Magnesium: 1.8–2.4 mEq/L
    e. Chloride: 95–108 mEq/L
    f. Phosphorus: 1.7–2.6 mEq/L; 2.5–4.5 mg/dL
  2. Signs and symptoms of hypo-hyperkalemia, hypo-hypernatremia, hypo-hypercalcemia
  3. Urine osmolality 50–1400 mOsm/L (range); 500–800 mOsm/L (average)
    Urine specific gravity: 1.010–1.030
  4. Urine electrolytes
    a. Potassium: 25–120 mEq/24 h
    b. Sodium: 40–220 mEq/24 h
    c. Calcium: 50–150 mg/24 h
    d. Chloride: 110–250 mEq/24 h
    Example: Urine sodium 20 mOsm/L 24 hr: body retaining sodium even if serum sodium is low. Commonly seen with CHF and cirrhosis of the liver.
  5. Vital signs (VS): pulse irregular
  6. ECG: changes with potassium, sodium, calcium, and magnesium imbalances
  7. Behavioral changes: potassium imbalance
  8. Drug therapy: diuretics, steroids, digitalis preparations, antibiotics
  9. Continuous GI suctioning: loss of major electrolytes

D. Acid-base balance assessment
  1. Arterial blood gases (ABGs)
    a. pH: <7.35, acidosis; >7.45, alkalosis
    b. $PaCO_2$: <35 mm Hg, respiratory alkalosis; >45 mm Hg, respiratory acidosis
    c. HCO_3: <24 mEq/L, metabolic acidosis; >28 mEq/L, metabolic alkalosis
       Base excess (BE): <−2, metabolic acidosis; >+2, metabolic alkalosis
  2. Serum CO_2: 22–32 mEq/L
  3. Overbreathing or underbreathing
  4. Chest sounds: rales, rhonchi
  5. Assisted ventilator
  6. Behavioral changes: acid-base imbalance present
  7. Intubations
  8. Electrolyte imbalance: loss of potassium (K) and hydrochloric acid (HCl): hypokalemic alkalosis

Appendix F

Foods Rich in Potassium, Sodium, Calcium, Magnesium, Chloride, and Phosphorous

Classes	Potassium	Sodium	Calcium	Magnesium	Chloride	Phosphorus
Daily requirements	3–4 g	2–4 g	800 mg	300–350 mg	3–9 g	800–1200 mg
Beverages	Cocoa, Coca-Cola, coffee, wines	Pepsi-Cola, tea, decaffeinated coffee		Cocoa		
Fruit and fruit juices	Citrus fruits: oranges, grapefruit Juices: grapefruit (canned), orange (canned), prune (canned), tomato (canned) Fruits: apricots (dry), bananas, cantaloupe, dates, raisins (dry), watermelon, prunes			Average	High only in dates and bananas	
Bread products and cereal	Average to low amount	White bread, soda crackers, and wheat flakes		Cereals with oats		Whole grain cereal
Dairy products	Average to low—milk, buttermilk	Butter, cheese, and margarine	Milk, cheese	Milk (average)	Cheese, milk	Cheese, milk, eggs
Nuts	Almonds, Brazil nuts, cashews, and peanuts	Low, except if salted	Brazil nuts (moderate)	Almonds, Brazil nuts, peanuts, and walnuts		Peanuts

(continued on the following page)

(Continued)

Classes	Potassium	Sodium	Calcium	Magnesium	Chloride	Phosphorus
Vegetables	Baked beans, carrots (raw), celery (raw), dandelion greens, lima beans (canned), mustard greens, tomatoes, spinach *Note:* Nearly all vegetables are rich in potassium when raw, but K will be lost if water used in cooking is discarded.	Average to low Celery (high average)	Baked beans, kale, mustard and turnip greens, broccoli	Green, leafy	Spinach, celery	Dry beans
Meat, fish, and poultry	Average—meats High average—sardines, codfish, scallops	Corned beef, bacon, ham, crab, tuna fish, sausage (pork) Low in poultry	Salmon, meats	Fish, shrimp Low in poultry Low in meats Egg, average	Eggs, crabs, fish (average), turkey	Beef, pork, fish, chicken, turkey
Miscellaneous	Catsup (average), spices, potato chips, and peanut butter	Catsup, mayonnaise, potato chips, pretzels, pickles, dill, olives, mustard, Worcestershire sauce, celery salt, salad dressing—French and Italian	Molasses	Chocolate and chocolate bars, chocolate syrup Molasses Table salt		

Appendix G

Common Laboratory Tests and Values for Adults and Children

Reference Values

Hematology	Color-Top Tube	Adult	Child
Bleeding time		Ivy's method: 3–7 minutes	Same as adult
Carboxyhemoglobin (CO)—See Chemistry.		Duke's method: 1–3 minutes	
Clot retraction	Red	1–24 h	Same as adult
Coagulation time (CT)		5–15 min	Same as adult
		Average: 8 min	
Erythrocyte sedimentation rate (ESR)	Lavender	<50 years old (Westergren)	Newborn:
		Male: 0–15 mm/h	0–2 mm/h
		Female: 0–20 mm/h	4–14 years old:
		>50 years old (Westergren)	0–10 mm/h
		Male: 0–20 mm/h	
		Female: 0–30 mm/h	
		Wintrobe method:	
		Male: 0–9 mm/h	
		Female: 0–15 mm/h	
Factor assay	Blue		
I Fibrinogen		200–400 mg/dL	Same as adult
		Minimum for clotting: 75–100 mg/dL	
II Prothrombin		Minimum hemostatic level: 10%–15% concentration	
III Thromboplastin		Variety of substances	
IV Calcium		4.5–5.5 mEq/L or 9–11 mg/dL	
V Proaccelerin labile factor		Minimum hemostatic level: 50%–150% activity;	Same as adult
		5%–10% concentration	
VI		Not used	
VII Proconvertin stable factor		Minimum hemostatic level: 65%–135% activity;	
		5%–15% concentration	
VIII Antihemophilic factor (AHF)		Minimum hemostatic level: 55%–145% activity;	
		30%–35% concentration	

IX Plasma thromboplastin component (PTC, Christmas factor)		Minimum hemostatic level: 60%–140% activity; 30% concentration
X Stuart factor, Prower factor		Minimum hemostatic level: 45%–150% activity; 7%–10% concentration
XI Plasma thromboplastin antecedent (PTA)		Minimum hemostatic level: 65%–135% activity; 20%–30% concentration
XII Hageman factor		0% concentration
XIII Fibrinase, fibrin stabilizing factor (FSF)		Minimum hemostatic level: 1% concentration
Fibrin degradation products (FDP)	Red	2–10 μg/mL
Fibrinogen	Blue	200–400 mg/dL
		Not usually done
		Newborn: 150–300 mg/dL
		Child: same as adult
Hematocrit (Hct)	Lavender	Male: 40%–54%; 0.40–0.54 SI units
		Female: 36%–46%; 0.36–0.46 SI units
		Newborn: 44%–65%
		1–3 years old: 29%–40%
		4–10 years old: 31%–43%
Hemoglobin (Hb or Hgb)	Lavender	Male: 13.5–17 g/dL
		Female: 12–15 g/dL
		Newborn: 14–24 g/dL
		Infant: 10–17 g/dL
		Child: 11–16 g/dL
Hemoglobin electrophoresis	Lavender	
A₁		95%–98% total Hb
A₂		1.5%–4.0%
F		<2%
		Newborn: 50%–80% total Hb
		Infant: 2%–8% total Hb
		Child: 1%–2% total Hb
C		0%
D		0%
S		0%
Lymphocytes (T & B) assay	Lavender (2 tubes)	T cells: 60%–80%, 600–2400 cells/μL
		B cells: 4%–16%, 50–250 cells/μL
Partial thromboplastin time (PTT)	Blue	PPT: 60–70 seconds
		APTT: 25–40 seconds
Plasminogen	Blue	2.5–5.2 U/mL
		3.8–8.4 CTA

(continued on the following page)

Hematology	Color-Top Tube	Reference Values	
		Adult	Child
Platelet aggregation and adhesion	Blue	Aggregation in 3–5 minutes	
Platelet count (thrombocytes)	Lavender	150,000–400,000 μL (mean, 250,000 μL)	Premature:
			100,000–300,000 μL
		SI units: 0.15–0.4 × 10^{12}/L	Newborn:
			150,000–300,000 μL
			Infant: 200,000–475,000 μL
			Same as adult
Prothrombin time (PT)	Blue or black	11–15 seconds or 70%–100%	
		Anticoagulant therapy: 2–2.5 times the control in seconds or	
		20%–30%	
RBC indices (mil/μL)	Lavender	Male: 4.6–6.0	Newborn: 4.8–7.2
		Female: 4.0–5.0	Child: 3.8–5.5
MCV (cuμ)		80–98	Newborn: 96–108
			Child: 82–92
MCH (pg)		27–31	Newborn: 32–34
			Child: 27–31
MCHC (%)		32–36	Newborn: 32–33
RDW (Coulter S)		11.5–14.5	Child: 32–36
Reticulocyte count	Lavender	0.5%–1.5% of all RBCs	Newborn: 2.5%–6.5% of all RBCs
			Infant: 0.5%–3.5% of all RBCs
		25,000–75,000 μL (absolute count)	Child: 0.5%–2.0% of all RBCs
Sickle cell screening	Lavender	0	0
White blood cells (WBC)	Lavender	4,500–10,000 μL	Newborn: 9,000–30,000 μL
			2 years old: 6,000–17,000 μL
			10 years: 4,500–13,500 μL

		Reference Values	
		Adult	**Child**
White blood cell differential	Lavender	50%–70% of total WBCs	29%–47%
Neutrophils		50%–65%	
Segments		0%–5%	
Bands		0%–3%	0%–3%
Eosinophils		1%–3%	1%–3%
Basophils		25%–35%	38%–63%
Lymphocytes		2%–6%	4%–9%
Monocytes			
Immunohematology (Blood Bank)			
Coombs direct	Lavender	Negative	Negative
Coombs indirect	Red	Negative	Negative
Cross matching	Red	Absence of agglutination (clumping)	Same as adult
Rh typing	Red	Rh+ and Rh−	Same as adult

Chemistry	**Color-Top Tube**	**Adult**	**Child**
Acetaminophen	Red	Therapeutic: 5–20 µg/mL; 31–124 µmol/L (SI units) Toxic: >50 µg/mL; >305 µmol/L (SI units) >200 µg/mL, possible hepatotoxicity	Therapeutic: same as adult
Acetone (ketone bodies)	Red	Acetone: 0.3–2.0 mg/dL; 51.6–344 µmol/L (SI units) Ketones: 2–4 mg/dL	Newborn: slightly higher than adult Infant and child: same as adult
Acid phosphatase (ACP)	Red	0.0–0.8 U/L at 37°C (SI units)	6.4–15.2 U/L
Adrenocorticotropic Hormone (ACTH)	Lavender	7–10 AM: 15–80 pg/mL; 4 PM: 5–30 pg/mL; 10 PM to Midnight: <10 pg/mL	
Alanine aminotransferase (ALT, SGPT)	Red	10–35 U/L	Same as adult Infant: could be twice as high
Albumin	Red	3.5–5 g/dL	
Alcohol	Red	0%	

(continued on the following page)

Reference Values

Chemistry	Color-Top Tube	Adult	Child
Aldolase (ALD)	Red	3–8 U/dL (Sibley-Lehninger)	Infant: 12–24 U/dL Child: 6–16 U/dL
Aldosterone	Red or green	22–59 mU/L at 37°C (SI units)	3–11 years: 5–70 mg/dL
Alkaline phosphatase (ALP)	Red	Fast: <16 mg/dL; 4–30 mg/dL (sitting position)	Infant: 40–300 U/L Child: 60–270 U/L
ALP[1]		41–136 U/L	
ALP[2]		20–130 U/L	Older child: 50–230 U/L
Alpha$_1$-antitrypsin	Red	20–120 U/L 78–200 mg/dL 0.78–2.0 g/L	Newborn: 145–270 mg/dL Infant and child: same as adult
Alpha-fetoprotein (AFP)	Red	*(see sub-table below)*	
Ammonia	Green	Toxic level: >500 ng/mL 15–45 µg/dL 11–35 µmol/L (SI units)	Newborn: 64–107 µg/dL Child: 21–50 µg/dL
Amylase		30–170 µ/L Isoenzymes: S: 45–70% P: 30–55%	
Angiotensin-converting enzyme (ACE)	Red or green	11–67 U/L	Not usually performed
Anion gap		10–17 mEq/L	
Antidiuretic hormone (ADH)	Lavender	1–5 pg/mL 1–5 ng/L	
Arterial blood gases (See *Others*)			

Alpha-fetoprotein (AFP):

Weeks of Gestation	Serum (ng/mL)	Amniotic Fluid (µg/mL)
14	7–50	11.0–32.0
15	7–60	5.5–31.0
16	10–72	5.7–31.5
17	11–90	3.8–32.5
18	14–94	3.6–28.0
19	24–112	3.7–24.5
20	31–122	2.2–15.0

Test	Tube	Adult value	Newborn/Child value
Ascorbic acid (vitamin C)	Gray or red	0.6–2.0 mg/dL (plasma)	0.6–1.6 mg/dL (plasma)
Aspartate aminotransferase	Red	34–114 μmol/L (SI units, plasma) 0.2–2.0 mg/dL (blood) 12–114 μmol (SI units, serum) 0–35 U/L	Newborn: four times normal level Child: same as adult
(AST, SGOT)		Average 8–38 U/L	
Bilirubin (indirect)	Red	0.1–1.0 mg/dL 1.7–17.1 μmol/L (SI units)	
Bilirubin (total and direct)	Red	Total: 0.1–1.2 mg/dL; 1.7–20.5 μmol/L (SI units)	Newborn, total: 1–12 mg/dL; 17.1–205 μmol/L (SI units) Child, total: 0.2–0.8 mg/dL
Blood urea nitrogen (BUN)	Red	Direct (conjugated): 0.1–0.3 mg/dL; 1.7–5.1 μmol/L (SI units) 5–25 mg/dL	Infant: 5–15 mg/dL Child: 5–20 mg/dL
BUN/creatinine ratio	Red	10:1 to 20:1	
Calcitonin	Green or lavender	Male: <40 pg/mL Female: <25 pg/mL	Newborn: usually higher Child: <70 pg/mL
Calcium (Ca)	Red	4.5–5.5 mEq/L 9–11 mg/dL 2.3–2.8 mmol/L (SI units)	Newborn: 3.7–7.0 mEq/L; 7.4–14 mg/dL Infant: 5.0–6.0 mEq/L; 10–12 mg/dL Child: 4.5–5.8 mEq/L; 9–11.5 mg/dL
Ionized calcium (iCa)		4.4–5.9 mg/dL 2.2–2.5 mEq/L 1.1–1.24 mmol/L	
Carbamazepine	Red	Therapeutic: 4–12 μg/mL; 16.9–50.8 μmol/L (SI units) Toxic: >12–15 μg/mL; >50.8–69 μmol/L (SI units)	
Carbon dioxide combining power (CO_2)	Green	22–30 mEq/L 22–30 mmol/L (SI units)	20–28 mEq/L
Carbon monoxide (CO)	Lavender	<2.5% saturation of Hb	Same as adult

(continued on the following page)

Chemistry	Color-Top Tube	Reference Values	
		Adult	Child
Carboxyhemoglobin (may be done in hematology)		2%–9% saturation of Hb (smokers)	
Carotene	Red	60–200 mg/dL	40–130 μg/dL
Catecholamines	Green or lavender	0.74–3.72 μmol/L (SI units)	
		Positive for pheochromocytoma: >1000 pg/mL	
Epinephrine		Supine: <50 pg/mL	
		Sitting: <60 pg/mL	
		Standing: <90 pg/mL	
Norepinephrine		Supine: 110–410 pg/mL	
		Sitting: 120–680 pg/mL	
		Standing: 125–700 pg/mL	
Dopamine		Supine and standing: <87 pg/mL	
Ceruloplasmin (Cp)	Red	18–45 mg/dL	Infant: <23 mg/dL or normal
			Child: 30–65 mg/dL
Chloride (Cl)	Red	180–450 mg/L (SI units)	Newborn: 94–112 mEq/L
		95–105 mEq/L	Infant: 95–110 mEq/L
		95–105 mmol/L (SI units)	Child: 98–105 mEq/L
Cholesterol	Red		Infant: 90–130 mg/dL
		Desirable level: <200 mg/dL	2–19 years:
		Moderate risk: 200–240 mg/dL	Desirable level: 130–170
		High risk: >240 mg/dL	mg/dL;
			Moderate risk: 171–84
			mg/dL; High risk: >185
			mg/dL
Cholinesterase	Green	0.5–1.0 U (RBC)	Same as adult
		3–8 U/mL (plasma)	
		6–8 IU/L (RBC)	
		8–18 IU/L at 37°C (plasma)	

Test	Tube	Values	
Copper (Cu)	Red or green	Male: 70–140 µg/dL; 11–22 µmol/L (SI units) Female: 80–155 µg/dL; 12.6–24.3 µmol/L (SI units) Pregnancy: 140–300 µg/dL	Newborn: 20–70 µg/dL Child: 30–190 µg/dL Adolescent: 90–240 µg/dL
Cortisol	Green	8 AM–10 AM: 5–23 µg/dL; 138–635 nmol/L (SI units) 4 PM–6 PM: 3–13 µg/dL; 83–359 nmol/L (SI units)	8 AM–10 AM: 15–25 µg/dL 4 PM–6 PM: 5–10 µg/dL
Creatinine phosphokinase (CPK)	Red	Male: 5–35 µg/mL; 30–180 IU/L, 55–170 U/L at 37°C (SI units) Female: 5–25 µg/mL; 25–150 IU/L; 30–135 U/L at 37°C (SI units)	Newborn: 65–580 IU/L at 30°C Child: Male: 0–70 IU/L at 30°C Female: 0–50 IU/L at 30°C
Creatinine	Red	0.5–1.5 mg/dL 45–132.3 µmol/L (SI units)	Newborn: 0.8–1.4 mg/dL Infant: 0.7–1.7 mg/dL 2–6 years: 0.3–0.6 mg/dL, 24–54 µmol/L (SI units) 7–18 years: 0.4–1.2 mg/dL, 36–106 µmol/L (SI units)
Cryoglobulins	Red	Negative	
Disseminated intravascular coagulation (DIC) screening test		See Part III, Hematologic Conditions.	
Dexamethasone suppression test	Green	Cortisol: 8 AM: <10 µg/dL	
Digoxin	Red	Therapeutic: 0.5–2 ng/mL; 0.5–2 nmol/L (SI units)	Therapeutic: Infant: 1–3 ng/mL; 1–3 nmol/L (SI units) Toxic: >3.5 ng/mL
D-xylose absorption	Red	Toxic: >2 ng/mL; >2.6 nmol/L (SI units) 25–40 mg/dL/2h Elderly: same as adult	30 mg/dL/1h

Estetrol (E₄) | Red

Pregnancy:

Weeks of Gestation	pg/mL
20–26	140–210
30	350
36	900
40	>1050

(continued on the following page)

Reference Values

Chemistry	Color-Top Tube	Adult	Child
Estradiol (E$_2$)	Red	Female: Follicular phase: 20–150 pg/mL Midcycle: 100–500 pg/mL Luteal: 60–260 pg/mL Postmenopausal: <30 pg/mL Male: 15–50 pg/mL Pregnancy:	3–10 pg/mL
Estriol/E$_3$	Red	**Serum** **Weeks of Gestation** — **ng/dL** 25–28: 25–165 29–32: 30–230 33–36: 45–370 37–38: 75–420 39–40: 95–450	
Estrone (E$_1$)	Red	Female: 2 Follicular phase: 30–100 pg/mL Ovulatory phase: >150 pg/mL Luteal phase: 90–160 pg/mL Postmenopausal: 20–40 pg/mL Male: 10–50 pg/mL	1–10 years: <10 pg/mL
Estrogen	Red	Female: Early menstrual cycle: 60–200 pg/mL Midcycle: 120–440 pg/mL Male: 40–155 pg/mL	1–6 years: 3–10 pg/mL 8–12 years: <30 pg/mL
Fasting blood sugar (FBS)	Gray or red	70–110 mg/dL (serum) 60–100 mg/dL (blood)	Newborn: 30–80 mg/dL Child: 60–100 mg/dL
Feasting blood sugar (*See Postprandial blood sugar.*)			

Test	Tube color	Adult values	Child values
Ferritin	Red	Female: 10–125 ng/mL 10–125 µg/L (SI units) Male: 35–300 ng/mL 35–300 µg/L (SI units)	Newborn: 20–200 ng/mL Infant: 30–200 ng/mL 1–16 years: 8–140 ng/mL
Folate (folic acid) (may be done by nuclear medicine)	Red	3–16 ng/mL (bioassay) >2.5 ng/mL (RIA, serum) 200–700 ng/mL (RBC)	Same as adult
Follicle-stimulating hormone (FSH)	Red	Pre/postovulation: 4–30 mU/mL Midcycle: 10–90 mU/mL Postmenopausal: 40–170 mU/mL Male: 4–25 mU/mL	5–12 mU/mL
Gamma-glutamyl transferase (GGT)	Red	Male: 4–23 IU/L Female: 3–13 IU/L; 4–33 U/L at 37°C (SI units)	
Gastrin	Red or lavender	Fasting: <100 pg/mL 8–18 IU/gHb	Not usually performed
Glucose-6-phosphate dehydrogenase (G-6-PD) (may be done in hematology)	Lavender or green	125–281 U/dL (packed RBC) 251–511 U/dL (cells) 1211–2111 mIU/mL (packed RBC)	Same as adult
Glucose—fasting blood sugar (See Fasting blood sugar.)	Lavender		
Glucagon	Gray or red	50–200 pg/mL	
Glucose tolerance test (GTT)		(see table below)	

Time	Serum (mg/dL)	Blood (mg/dL)	Child (6 years or older)
Fasting	70–110	60–100	Same as adult
0.5 hour	<160	<150	
1 hour	<170	<160	
2 hour	<125	<115	
3 hour	Fasting level	Fasting level	

Test	Tube color	Values
Growth hormone	Red	Male: <5 ng/mL Female: <10 ng/mL / <10 ng/mL

(continued on the following page)

Chemistry	Color-Top Tube	Reference Values	
		Adult	Child
Hexosaminidase	Red	Total: 5–20 U/L A: 55%–80%	
Human chorionic gonadotropin (HCG)	Red	Nonpregnant female: <0.01 IU/mL **Pregnant (Weeks)** **Values** 1 0.01–0.04 IU/mL 2 0.03–0.10 IU/mL 4 0.10–1.0 IU/mL 5–12 10–100 IU/mL 13–25 10–30 IU/mL 26–40 5–15 IU/mL	
Human immunosuppressive virus (HIV)	Red	Negative	
Human leukocyte antigen (HLA)	Green	Histocompatibility match	
Human placental lactogen (HPL)	Red or green	**Weeks of Gestation** **ng/mL** 8–27 4.6 μg/mL 28–31 2.4–6.0 μg/mL 32–35 3.7–7.7 μg/mL 36–40 5.0–10.0 μg/mL	
Immunoglobulins (See Serology.)	Red		
Insulin	Red	5–25 μU/mL	
Iron	Red	50–150 μg/dL; 10–27 μmol/L (SI units)	
Iron-binding capacity (IBC, TIBC)	Red	250–450 μg/dL	Infant (6 months–2 years): 40–100 μg/dL Newborn: 100–270 μg/dL Infant (6 months–2 years): 100–350 μg/dL Child: same as adult

Test	Tube color	Values	
Lactic acid	Green	Arterial blood: 0.5–2.0 mEq/L; <11.3 mg/dL; Venous blood: 0.5–1.5 mEq/L; 8.1–15.3 mg/dL; Critical: >5 mEq/L; >45 mg/dL	
Lactic dehydrogenase (LDH/LD)	Red	100–190 IU/L; 70–250 U/L	Newborn: 300–1500 IU/L; Child: 50–150 IU/L
LDH isoenzymes	Red		
LDH$_1$		14%–26%	
LDH$_2$		27%–37%	
LDH$_3$		13%–26%	
LDH$_4$		8%–16%	
LDH$_5$		6%–16%	
Lactose tolerance test	Gray	20–50 mg/dL rise from fasting blood glucose	
Lead	Lavender or green	10–20 µg/dL; 20–40 µg/dL (acceptable)	10–20 µg/dL; 20–30 µg/dL (acceptable)
LE cells (Lupus) also in hematology	Red or green	Negative	
Lecithin/sphingomyelin ratio (L/S; amniotic fluid)		1:1 before 35 weeks of gestation; L: 6–9 mg/dL; S: 4–6 mg/dL; 4:1 after 35 weeks of gestation; L: 15–21 mg/dL; S: 4–6 mg/dL	
Leucine aminopeptidase (LAP)	Red	8–22 mU/mL, 12–33 IU/L; 75–200 U/mL	Infant: 9–105 IU/L at 37°C; Child: 20–136 IU/L at 37°C
Lipase	Red	20–180 IU/L; 14–280 mU/mL; 14–280 U/L (SI units)	
Lipoproteins (*See Cholesterol, Phospholipids, and Triglycerides.*)			
Lithium	Red	0; Therapeutic: 0.8–1.2 mEq/L; Toxic: >2 mEq/L	0

(continued on the following page)

Reference Values

Chemistry	Color-Top Tube	Adult	Child
Luteinizing hormone (LH)	Red or lavender	Pre/postovulation: 5–30 mIU/mL Midcycle: 50–150 mIU/mL Postmenopause: >35 mIU/mL Male: 5–25 mIU/mL	6–12 years: <10 mIU/mL 13–18 years: <20 mIU/mL
Magnesium (Mg)	Red	1.5–2.5 mEq/L; 1.8–3.0 mg/dL	Newborn: 1.4–2.9 mEq/L Child: 1.6–2.6 mEq/L
Myoglobin	Red	12–90 μg/L; 12–90 ng/mL	
Nifedipine	Red	Therapeutic: 50–100 ng/mL Toxic: >100 ng/mL Toxic level: >200 ng/mL	
5'Nucleotidase (5'N)	Red	<17 U/L	
Osmolality	Red	280–300 mOsm/kg	270–290 mOsm/kg
Parathyroid hormone (PTH)	Red	PTH: 11–54 pg/mL C Terminal PTH: 50–330 pg/mL; N-Terminal PTH: 8–24 pg/mL	
Pepsinogen I	Red	124–142 ng/mL	Premature: 20–24 ng/mL <1 year: 72–82 ng/mL 1–2 years: 90–106 ng/mL 3–6 years: 80–104 ng/mL 7–10 years: 77–103 ng/mL 11–14 years: 96–118 ng/mL
Phospholipids	Red	150–380 mg/dL	
Phosphorus (P) (inorganic)	Red	1.7–2.6 mEq/L 2.5–4.5 mg/dL	Newborn: 3.5–8.6 mg/dL Infant: 4.5–6.7 mg/dL Child: 4.5–5.5 mg/dL
Postprandial blood sugar (feasting: PPBS)	Gray or red	<140 mg/dL 2 hours (plasma) <120 mg/dL 2 hours (blood) Older adult: <160 mg/dL 2 hours (plasma); <140 mg/dL 2 hours (blood)	Same as adult

Potassium (K)	Red	3.5–5.3 mEq/L	Infant: 3.6–5.8 mEq/L
		3.5–5.3 mmol/L (SI units)	Child: 3.5–5.5 mEq/L
Progesterone	Red	Female:	
		Follicular phase: 0.1–1.5 ng/mL	
		Luteal: 2–28 ng/mL	
		Pregnancy:	
		First trimester: 9–50 ng/mL	
		Second trimester: 18–150 ng/mL	
		Third trimester: 60–260 ng/mL	
		Male: <1.0 ng/mL	
Prolactin (PRL)	Red or lavender	Nonpregnant:	
		Follicular phase: 0–23 ng/mL	
		Luteal: 0–40 ng/mL	
		Postmenopausal: <12 ng/mL	
		Pregnancy:	
		First trimester: <80 ng/mL	
		Second trimester: <160 ng/mL	
		Third trimester: <400 ng/mL	
		Male: 0.1–20 ng/mL	
		Pituitary adenoma: >100–300 ng/mL	
Prostate-specific antigen (PSA)	Red	Normal: 0–4 ng/mL	
		BPH: 4–19 ng/mL	
		Prostate cancer:	
		10–120 ng/mL	
Protein	Red	6.0–8.0 g/dL	Premature: 4.2–7.6 g/dL
			Newborn: 4.6–7.4 g/dL
			Infant: 6.0–6.7 g/dL
			Child: 6.2–8.0 g/dL

(continued on the following page)

Chemistry	Color-Top Tube	Reference Values	
		Adult	**Child**
Protein electrophoresis	Red	Albumin: 3.5–5.0 g/dL; 52%–68% of total protein	Premature: 3.0–4.2 g/dL Newborn: 3.5–5.4 g/dL Infant: 4.4–5.4 g/dL Child: 4.0–5.8 g/dL
Renin	Lavender	Globulin: 1.5–3.5 g/dL; 32%–48% of total protein Normal sodium diet: supine: 0.2–2.3 ng/mL; upright: 1.6–4.3 ng/mL. Restricted salt diet: upright: 4.1–10.8 ng/mL	3–5 years: 1.0–6.5 ng/mL 5–10 years: 0.5–6.0 ng/mL

Salicylate	Red	0
		Therapeutic: 15–30 mg/dL
		Toxic:
		  Mild: >30 mg/dL
		  Severe: >50 mg/dL
			0
			Toxic: >25 mg/dL

Serotonin	Lavender	50–175 ng/mL; 10–30 µg/dL; 0.29–1.15 µmol/L (SI units)	
Sodium (Na)	Red	135–145 mEq/L 135–142 nmol/L (SI units)	Infant: 134–150 mEq/L Child: 135–145 mEq/L
T₃	Red	80–200 ng/dL	Newborn: 90–170 ng/dL Child, 6–12 years: 115–190 ng/dL
Testosterone	Red or green	Male: 0.3–1.0 µg/dL; 300–1000 ng/dL Female: 0.03–0.1 µg/dL; 30–100 ng/dL	Male adolescent: >0.1 µg/dL Male, 12–14 years old: >100 ng/dL

Theophylline	Red	Therapeutic:
		  Adult: 5–20 µg/mL; 28–112 µmol/L (SI units)
		  Elderly: 5–18 µg/mL
		Toxic:
		  Adult: >20 µg/mL; >112 µmol/L (SI units)
		  Elderly: same as adult
			Therapeutic:
			  Premature: 7–14 µg/mL
			  Neonate: 3–12 µg/mL
			  Child: same as adult
			Toxic:
			  Premature: >14 µg/mL
			  Neonate: >13 µg/mL
			  Child: same as adult

Test	Tube	Values
Thyroid-binding globulin (TBG)	Red or green	10–26 µg/dL
Thyroxine (T_4)	Red	4.5–11.5 µg/dL (T_4 by column) 5–12 µg/dL (T_4 RIA) 1.0–2.3 ng/dL (Thyroxine iodine)	Newborn: 11–23 µg/dL 1–4 months: 7.5–16.5 µg/dL 4–12 months: 5.5–14.5 µg/dL 1–6 years: 5.5–13.5 µg/dL 6–10 years: 5–12.5 µg/dL Newborn: 125–275 mg/dL
Transferrin	Red	200–430 mg/dL; 2–4.3 g/L (SI units) Pregnancy (full term): 300 mg/dL
Transferrin percent saturation	Red	Male: 30%–50% Female: 20%–35%
T_3 resin uptake (may be done by nuclear medicine)	Red	25–35 relative % uptake	Not usually done
Tricyclic antidepressants		
Triglycerides	Red	10–150 mg/dL 0.11–2.09 mmol/L (SI units)	Infant: 5–40 mg/dL Child: 10–135 mg/dL
Uric acid	Red	Male: 3.5–8.0 mg/dL Female: 2.8–6.8 mg/dL	2.5–5.5 mg/dL
Vancomycin	Red	Therapeutic range: Peak: 20–40 µg/mL Trough: 5–10 µg/mL Toxic level: >40 µg/mL
Vitamin A	Red	30–95 µg/dL; 1.05–3.0 µmol/L (SI units); 125–150 IU/dL	1–6 years: 20–43 µg/dL; 0.7–1.5 µmol/L (SI units) 7–12 years: 26–50 µg/dL 13–19 years: 26–72 µg/dL
Vitamin B_1	Red	10–60 ng/mL; 5.3–8.0 µg/dL	
Vitamin B_6	Lavender	5–30 ng/mL; 20–120 nmol/L (SI units)	
Vitamin B^{12}	Red	200–900 pg/mL	
Vitamin C (See *Ascorbic acid*)			
Vitamin D_3	Red or green	1,23 dihydroxy: 20–76 pg/mL 25-hydroxy: 10–55 ng/mL	Newborn: 160–1200 pg/mL

(continued on the following page)

Chemistry	Color-Top Tube	Reference Values	
		Adult	**Child**
Vitamin E	Red	5–20 µg/mL; 0.5–1.8 mg/dL; 12–42 µmol/L (SI units)	3–15 µg/mL; 0.3–1.0 mg/dL; 7–23 µmol/L (SI units)
Zinc	Navy-blue	60–150 µg/dL 11–23 µmol/L (SI units)	
Zinc	Urine	150–1250 µg/24 h	
Zinc protoporphyrin (ZPP)	Green or lavender	15–77 µg/dL Average: <35 µg/dL; <0.56 µmol/L (SI units)	Same as adult

Serology	Color-Top Tube	Reference Values	
		Adult	**Child**
Adenovirus antibody	Red	Negative	Negative
Anti-DNA	Red	<1:85	<1:60
Antiglomerular basement membrane antibody (AGBM)	Red	Negative	<1:70
Antimitochondrial antibody (AMA)	Red	Negative at 1:5 Positive: >1:160	
Antimyocardial antibody	Red	None detected	
Antinuclear antibodies (ANA)	Red	Negative at 1:20 dilution	
Antistreptolysin O (ASO)	Red	100 IU/mL; <160 Todd U/mL	Negative Newborn: similar to mother's 2–5 years: <100 IU/mL 12–19 years: <200 IU/mL; <200 Todd U/mL

Carcinoembryonic antigen (CEA) (may be done by nuclear medicine)	Red or lavender	<2.5 ng/mL (nonsmokers) <3.5 ng/mL (smokers)	Not usually done
Chlamydia test	Red	<1:16	Same as adult
Cold agglutinins (CA)	Red	1:8 antibody titer	Not usually done
Complement (total)	Red	75–160 U/mL; 75–160 kU/L (SI units)	
Complement C_3	Red	Male: 80–180 mg/dL; 0.8–1.8 g/L (SI units) Female: 76–120 mg/dL; 0.76–1.2 g/L (SI units)	Not usually done
Complement C_4	Red	15–45 mg/dL; 150–450 mg/L (SI units)	Not usually done
C-reactive protein (CRP)	Red	0	0
Cryoglobulins	Red	Up to 6 mg/dL	Negative
Cytomegalovirus (CMV) antibody	Red	Negative to <0.30	
Encephalitis virus antibody	Red	Titer: <1:10	
Enterovirus group	Red	Negative	
Febrile agglutinins	Red	Febrile group: titers *Brucella:* <1:20 *Tularemia:* <1:40 *Salmonella:* <1:40 *Proteus:* <1:40	Same as adult
FTA-ABS (fluorescent treponemal antibody absorption)	Red	Negative	Negative
Haptoglobin	Red	60–270 mg/dL 0.6–2.7 g/L (SI units)	Newborn: 0–10 mg/dL Infant: 1–6 months: 0–30 mg/dL, then gradual increase
HB_s Ab	Red	Negative	Negative
HB_c Ab	Red	Negative	Negative
Hepatitis A virus (HAV)	Red	None detected	
Hepatitis B surface antigen (HB_sAg)	Red	Negative	Negative
Herpes simplex virus (HSV)	Red	<1:10	
Heterophile antibody	Red	<1:28 titer	Same as adult

(continued on the following page)

Reference Values

Serology	Color-Top Tube	Adult	Child	
			1–3 years old	*7–11 years old*
Immunoglobulins (Ig)	Red			
Total Ig		900–2200 mg/dL	400–1500 mg/dL	700–1700 mg/dL
IgG		800–1800 mg/dL	300–1400 mg/dL	600–1450 mg/dL
IgA		100–400 mg/dL	20–150 mg/dL	50–200 mg/dL
IgM		50–150 mg/dL	20–100 mg/dL	30–120 mg/dL
IgD		0.5–3 mg/dL		
Legionnaire antibody test	Red	Negative	Same as adult	
Lyme antibody test	Red	Titer <1:256		
Mumps antibody	Red	Negative or <1:8 titer		
Rabies antibody test	Red	IFA: <1:16		
Rapid plasma reagin (RPR)	Red	Negative	Negative	
Rhematoid factory (RF)	Red	<1:20 titer	Not usually done	
Rubella antibody detection (HAI or HI)	Red	<1:8 titer susceptible / 1:10–1:32 titer, past rubella exposure / 1:32–1:64 titer, immunity / >1:64 titer, definite immunity	Same as adult	
Thyroid antibodies (TA)	Red	Negative or <1:20 titer	Not usually done	
TORCH test	Red	Negative	Negative	
Toxoplasmosis antibody test	Red	No infection: <1:4 / Infected: >1:256		
Venereal disease research laboratory (VDRL)	Red	Negative	Negative	

Reference Values

Urine Chemistry	Adult	Child
Aldosterone	6–25 µg/24 h	Not usually done
Amylase	4–37 U/L/2h	Not usually done

Test	Value	Pediatric
Ascorbic acid tolerance (4-, 5-, or 6-hour sample)	Oral: 10% of administered amount IV: 30%–40% of administered amount	Not usually done
Bilirubin and bile	Negative to 0.02 mg/dL	Same as adult
Calcium (Ca)	100–250 mg/24 h (average calcium diet) 2.50–6.25 mmol/24 h	Same as adult
Catecholamines	<100 µg/24 h <0.59 µmol/24h (SI units)	Lower level than adult—weight difference
Epinephrine	0–14 µg/dL (random)	
Norepinephrine	<20 ng/24 h	
Cortisol	<100 ng/24 h	
Creatinine clearance	24–105 µg/24 h	
Creatinine	85–135 mL/min Male: 20–26 mg/kg/24 h; 0.18–0.23 mmol/kg/24 h (SI units) Female: 14–22 mg/kg/24 h; 0.12–0.19 mmol/kg/24 h (SI units)	Similar to adult
Estriol (E_3)	**Pregnant:**	

Weeks of Gestation	mg/24 h
25–28	6–28
29–32	6–32
33–36	10–45
37–40	15–60

Test	Value	Pediatric
Estrogens (total)	Female: Preovulation: 5–25 µg/24 h Follicular phase: 24–100 µg/24 h Luteal phase (menstruation): 22–80 µg/24 Postmenopause: 0–10 µg/24 h Male: 4–25 µg/24 h	<12 years: 1 µg/24h >12 years: same as adult
Estrone (E_1)	Female: Follicular phase: 4–7 µg/24 h Ovulatory phase: 11–30 µg/24 h Luteal phase: 10–22 µg/24 h Postmenopausal: 1–7 µg/24 h	

(continued on the following page)

Reference Values

Urine Chemistry	Adult	Child
Follicle-stimulating hormone (FSH)	Follicular: 2–15 IU/24 h Luteal phase: 4–20 IU/24 h Menopause: >50 IU/24 h	<10 mUU/24 h (prepubertal)
Human chorionic gonadotropin (HCG)	Positive for pregnancy: no agglutination Negative for pregnancy: agglutination	Not usually performed
17-Hydroxycorticosteroids (17-OHCS)	Male: 3–12 mg/24 h Female: 2–10 mg/24 h	Infant: <1 mg/24 h 2–4 years: 1–2 mg/24 h 5–12 years: 2–6 mg/24 h
5-Hydroxyindolacetic acid (5-HIAA)	Random: negative 24 hours: 2–10 mg/24 h	Not usually performed
Ketone bodies (acetone)	Negative	Negative

17-Ketosteroids (17-KS)	Male: 5–25 mg/24 h
	Female: 5–15 mg/24 h
	>65 years: 4–8 mg/24 h
		Infant: 1 mg/24 h
		1–3 years: <2 mg/24 h
		3–6 years: <3 mg/24 h
		7–10 years: <4 mg/24 h
		10–12 years:
		   Male: <6 mg/24 h
		   Female: <5 mg/24 h
		Adolescent:
		   Male: <3–15 mg/24 h
		   Female: <3–12 mg/24 h

Myoglobin	None detected	
Osmolality	50–1200 mOsm/kg Average: 200–800 mOsm/kg	Newborn: 100–600 mOsm/kg Child: same as adult

Phenylketonuria (PKU)	Not usually done	PKU: negative (positive when serum
		   phenylalanine is 12–15 mg/dL)
		Guthrie: negative (positive when serum
		   phenylalanine is 4 mg/dL)

Porphobilinogen	Random: negative 24 hour: 0–2 mg/24 h	Same as adult

Porphyrins	
Coproporphyrins	Random: 3–20 µg/dL 24 hours: 50–160 µg	0–80 µg/24 h
Uroporphyrins	Random: negative, 24 hours: <30 µg	10–30 µg/24 h 17–57 mEq/24 h
Potassium (K)	25–120 mEq/24 h 25–120 mmol/24 h (SI units)	
Pregnanediol	Male: 0.1–1.5 mg/24 h	0.4–1.0 mg/24 h
	Female: 0.5–1.5 mg/24 h (proliferative phase); 2–7 mg/24 h (luteal phase); 0.1–1.0 mg/24 h (postmenopausal)	

Pregnancy:

Gestation Weeks	mg/24 h
10–19	5–25
20–28	15–42
29–32	25–49

Pregnanetriol	Male: 0.4–2.4 mg/24 h Female: 0.5–2.0 mg/24 h	Infant: 0–0.2 mg/24 h Child: 0–1.0 mg/24 h
Protein	0–5 mg/dL24 h	Same as adult
Sodium (Na)	40–220 mEq/24 h	Same as adult
Uric acid	250–500 mg/24 h (low-purine diet)	
Urinalysis		
pH	4.5–8.0	Newborn: 5–7 Child: 4.5–8
Specific gravity (SG)	1.005–1.030	Newborn: 1.001–1.020 Child: Same as adult
Protein	Negative	Negative
Glucose	Negative	Negative
Ketones	Negative	Negative
RBC	1–2/low-power field	Rare
WBC	3–4	0–4
Casts	Occasional hyaline	Rare
Vitamin B₁	100–200 µg/24 h	

(continued on the following page)

Reference Values

Others	Adult	Child
Urobilinogen	Random: 0.3–3.5 mg/dL	Same as adult
	0.05–2.5 mg/24 h	
	0.5–4.0 Ehrlich units/24 h	
	0.09–4.23 µmol/24 h (SI units)	
Bleeding time	Ivy's method: 3–7 minutes	Same as adult
Arterial blood gases (ABGs)		
pH	7.35–7.45	7.36–7.44
$PaCO_2$	35–45 mm Hg	Same as adult
PaO_2	75–100 mm Hg	Same as adult
HCO_3	24–28 mEq/L	Same as adult
BE	+2 to −2 (± 2 mEq/L)	Same as adult
Cerebrospinal fluid (CSF)		
Pressure	75–175 mm H_2O	50–100 mm H_2O
Cell count	0–8 mm³	0–8 mm³
Protein	15–45 mg/dL	15–45 mg/dL
Chloride	118–132 mEq/L	120–128 mEq/L
Glucose	40–80 mg/dL	35–75 mg/dL
Culture	No organism	No organism
	<60 mEq/L	<50 mEq/L
Chloride (sweat)	60–150 millim/mL	Not usually done
Semen examination	Volume: 1.5–5.0 mL	
	Morphology: >75% mature spermatozoa	
	Motility: >60% actively mobile spermatozoa	

From *Laboratory and Diagnostic Tests with Nursing Implications* (5th ed.), by J. L. Kee, 1999, Stamford, CT: Appleton & Lange. Copyright 1999 by Appleton & Lange. Reprinted with permission.

References/Bibliography

Abraham, W. T., & Schriert, R. W. (1994). Body fluid volume regulation in health and disease. *Advances in Internal Medicine, 39.* St. Louis: Mosby-Year Book Inc., pp. 23–43.

American Nurses Association. (1991). *Standards of clinical nursing practice.* Kansas City: Author.

Barone, M. A. (Ed.). (1996). *The Harriet Lane handbook* (14th ed.). St. Louis: Mosby.

Beckwith, N. (1987). Fundamentals of fluid resuscitation. *Nursing Life, 2*(3), 51–55.

Bezerra, J. A., Stathos, T. H., Duncan, B., Gaines, J. A., & Udall, J. N. (1992). Treatment of infants with acute diarrhea: What's recommended and what's practiced. *Pediatrics, 90,* 1–4.

Birney, M. H., & Penney, D. G. (1990). Atrial natriuretic peptide: A hormone with implications for clinical practice. *Heart and Lung, 19*(2), 174–182.

Bove, L. A. (1994). How fluids and electrolytes shift after surgery. *Nursing 1994, 24*(8), 34–39.

Brensilver, J. M., & Goldberger, E. (1996). *A primer of water, electrolyte, and acid-base syndromes* (8th ed.). Philadelphia: Davis.

Brown, R. G. (1993). Disorders of water and sodium balance. *Postgraduate Medicine, 93*(4), 227, 228, 231–234, 239–244.

Butts, E. E. (1987). Fluid and electrolyte disorders associated with diabetic ketoacidosis and hyperglycemic hyperosmolar nonketotic coma. *Nursing Clinics of North America, 22*(4), 827–836.

Cannon, P. J. (1989). Sodium retention in heart failure. *Cardiology Clinics, 7*(1), 49–59.

Carpentito, L. J. (1997). *Nursing diagnosis application to clinical practice* (7th ed.). Philadelphia: Lippincott.

Cefalu, W. T. (1991). Diabetic ketoacidosis. *Critical Care Clinics, 7*(1), 89–107.

Chambers, J. K. (1987). Fluid and electrolyte problems in renal and urologic disorders. *Nursing Clinics of North America, 22*(4), 815–825.

Chernow, B., Bamberger, E., & Stoiko, M. (1989). Hypomagnesemia in patients in postoperative intensive care. *Chest, 95*(2), 391–396.

Clark, B. A., & Brown, R. S. (1995). Potassium homeostasis and hyperkalemic syndromes. *Endocrinology and Metabolism Clinics of North America, 24*(3), 573–591.

Cornell, S. (1997). Maintaining a fluid balance. *Advance for Nurse practitioners, 5*(12), 43–44.

Davis, K. D., & Attie, M. F. (1991). Management of severe hypercalcemia. *Critical Care Clinics, 7*(1), 175–189.

Doran, A. (1992). S.I.A.D.D.: Is your patient at risk? *Nursing 92, 22*(6), 60–63.

Ebersole, P., & Hess, P. (1998). *Toward healthy aging: Human needs and nursing response* (5th ed.). Baltimore, MD: Mosby.

Felver, L., & Pendarvis, J. H. (1989). Electrolyte imbalances. *AORN Journal, 49*(4), 992–1005.

Foster, E. E., & Lefor, A. T. (1996). General management of gastrointestinal fistulas. *Surgical Clinics of North America, 76*(5), 1019–1033.

Freeman, B. I., & Burkart, J. M. (1991). Hypokalemia. *Critical Care Clinics, 7*(1), 143–153.

Fundamentals of fluid and electrolyte imbalances. (1982). Travenol Laboratories, Parenteral Products, Deerfield, IL.

German, K. (1987). Fluid and electrolyte problems associated with diabetes insipidus and syndrome of inappropriate antidiuretic hormone. *Nursing Clinics of North America, 22*(4), 785–795.

Gershan, J. A., Freeman, C. M., Ross, M. C., & members of the Research committee, Greater Milwaukee area chapter of the American Association of Critical Care Nurses. (1990). *Heart and Lung, 19*(2), 152–156.

Giesecke, A. H., Grande, C. M., & Whitten, C. W. (1990). Fluid therapy and the resuscitation of traumatic shock. *Critical Care Clinics, 6*(1), 61–71.

Guyton, A. C., & Hall, J. (1995). *Textbook of medical physiology* (9th ed.). Philadelphia: Saunders.

Hecker, J. (1988). Improve techniques in IV therapy. *Nursing Times, 84*(34), 28–33.

Heitkemper, M. M., & Bond, E. (1988). Fluid and electrolytes: Assessment and interventions. *Journal of Enterostomal Therapy, 15*(1), 18–23.

Held, J. L. (1995). Correcting fluid and electrolyte imbalance. *Nursing 1995, 25*(4), 71.

Hollifield, J. W. (1989). Electrolyte disarray and cardiovascular disease. *American Journal of Cardiology, 63,* 21B–26B.

Innerarity, S., & Stark, J. (1997). *Fluid and electrolytes.* Springhouse, PA.: Springhouse.

Intravenous Nurses's Society. (1998). *Intravenous nursing standards of practice.* Belmont, ME: Author.

Jones, A. M., Moseley, M. J., Halfmann, S. J., Heath, A. H., & Henkelman, N. J. (1991). Fluid volume dynamics. *Critical Care Nurse, 11*(4), 74–76.

Jones, D. H. (1991). Fluid therapy in the PACU. *Critical Care Nursing Clinics of North America, 3*(1), 109–130.

Kamel, K. S., Ethier, J. H., & Richardson, M. A. (1990). Urine electrolytes and osmolality: When and how to use them. *American Journal of Nephrology, 10*(2), 89–102.

Kamel, K. S., Magner, P. O. C., Ethier, J. H., & Halperin, M. L. (1989). Urine electrolytes in the assessment of extracellular fluid volume contraction. *American Journal of Nephrology, 9*(4), 344–347.

Karb, V. B. (1989). Electrolyte abnormalities and drugs which commonly cause them. *Journal of Neuroscience Nursing, 21*(2), 125–128.

Karch, A. (1998). *Nursing Drug Guide.* Philadelphia: Lippincott.

Kee, J. L. (1987). Potassium imbalance. *Nursing 1987, 17*(9), 32 K, M, P.

Kee, J. L. (1998). *Laboratory and diagnostic tests with nursing implications* (5th ed.). Stamford, CT: Appleton and Lange.

Kee, J. L., & Boyda, E. K. (1998). Knowledge base for patients with fluid, electrolyte, and acid-base imbalances. In F. D. Monahan, & M. Neighbors, *Surgical Nursing* (2nd ed., pp. 75–112). Philadelphia: Saunders.

Keyes, J. L. (1974). Blood-gas and blood-gas transport. *Heart and Lung, 3*(6), 945–954.

Keyes, J. L. (1976). Blood-gas analysis and the assessment of acid-base status. *Heart and Lung, 5*(2), 247–255.

Kleihenz, T. J. (1985). Preload and afterload. *Nursing 1985, 15*(5), 50–55.

Klemm, P. (1992). *Total nutritional admixture (TNA): Programmed instruction.* Baltimore: Johns Hopkins Hospital Department of Nursing.

Kokko, J. P., & Tanner, R. L. (1995). *Fluids and electrolytes* (3rd ed.). Philadelphia: Saunders.

Kositzke, J. A. (1990). A question of balance, dehydration in the elderly. *Journal of Gerontologic Nursing, 16*(5), 4–11, 40–41.

Lancaster, L. E. (1987a). *Core curriculum for nephrology nursing.* Pitman, NJ: Jannetti, Anthony J.

Lancaster, L. E. (1987b). Renal and endocrine regulation of water and electrolyte balance. *Nursing Clinics of North America, 22*(4), 761–772.

Lancour, J. (1978). ADH and aldosterone: How to recognize their effects. *Nursing 1978, 8*(9), 36–41.

Levy, D. B., & Peppers, M. P. (1991). IV fluids used in shock. *Emergency, 23*(4), 22–26.

Lorenz, J. M. (1997). Assessing fluid and electrolyte status in the newborn. *Clinical Chemistry, 43*(1), 205–210.

Lueckenotte, A. (1996). *Gerontologic nursing.* St. Louis: Mosby.

Martin, R. Y., & Schrier, R. W. (1995). Renal sodium excretion and edematous disorders. *Endocrinology and Metabolism Clinics of North America, 24*(3), 459–475.

Mathenson, M. (1989). Intravenous therapy. *Critical Care Nurse, 9*(2), 21–34.

Matz, R. (1994). Parallels between treated uncontrolled diabetes and the refeeding syndrome with emphasis on fluid and electrolyte abnormalities. *Diabetes Care, 17*(10), 1209–1213.

McCance, K., & Huether, S. (1990). *Pathophysiology: The biologic basis for disease in adults and children.* St. Louis: Mosby.

McConnell, E. A. (1987). Fluid and electrolyte concerns in intestinal surgical procedures. *Nursing Clinics of North America, 22*(4), 853–859.

310 ● References/Bibliography

McDermott, K. C., Almadrones, L. A., & Bajorunas, D. R. (1991). The diagnosis and management of hypomagnesemia: A unique treatment approach and case report. *Oncology Nursing Forum, 18,* 1145–1152.

McFadden, M. E., & Gatoricos, S. E. (1992). Multiple systems organ failure in the patient with cancer, Part I: Pathophysiologic perspectives. *Oncology Nursing Forum, 19,* 719–727.

Meador, B. (1982). Cardiogenic shock. *RN, 45*(4), 38–42.

Medical Center of Delaware. (1992). *Calculating infusion rate.* Newark, DE: Medical Center Orientation Materials.

Metheny, N. (1996). *Fluid and electrolyte balance* (3rd ed.). Philadelphia: Lippincott.

Meyers, K. A., & Hickey, M. K. (1988). Nursing management of hypovolemic shock. *Critical Care Nursing Quarterly, 11*(1), 57–67.

Millam, D. (1991). Myths and facts . . . About IV therapy. *Nursing 91, 21*(6), 75–76.

Miller, C. A. (1990). *Nursing care of older adults: Theory and practice.* Glenview, IL: Scott Foresman/Little, Brown.

Moiser, L. C. (1991). Anaphylaxis: A preventable complication of home infusion therapy. *Journal of Intravenous Nursing, 14*(2), 108–112.

Mueller, K. D., & Boisen, A. M. (1989). Keeping your patient's water level up. *RN, 52*(7), 65–68.

Nanji, A. (1983). Drug-induced electrolyte disorder. *Drug Intelligence and Clinical Pharmacy, 17,* 175–185.

Narins, R. G. (1982). Diagnostic strategies in disorders of fluid, electrolyte and acid-base homeostasis. *American Journal of Medicine, 72,* 496–518.

Norris, M. K. (1989). Dialysis disequilibrium syndrome. Action stat! *Nursing 1989, 19*(4), 33.

O'Donnell, M. E. (1995). Assessing fluid and electrolyte balance in elders. *American Journal of Nursing, 95*(11), 40–45.

Olinger, M. L. (1989). Disorders of calcium and magnesium metabolism. *Emergency Medicine Clinics of North America, 7*(4), 795–819.

Oster, J. R. Reston, R. A., & Materson, B. J. (1994). Fluid and electrolyte disorders in congestive heart failure. *Seminar Nephrology, 14*(5), 485–505.

Peppers, M. P., Geheb, M., & Desai, T. (1991). Hypophosphatemia and hyperphosphatemia. *Critical Care Clinics, 7*(1), 201–213.

Perkin, R., & Levin, D. L. (1980). Common fluid and electrolyte problems in the pediatric intensive care unit. *Pediatric Clinics of North America, 27*(3), 567–586.

Poe, C. M., & Radford, A. L. (1985). The challenge of hypercalcemia in cancer. *Oncology Nursing Forum, 12*(6), 29–34.

Porth, C. M. (1998). *Pathophysiology* (3rd ed.). Philadelphia: Lippincott.

Practice parameter: The management of acute gastroenteritis in young children. (1996). *Pediatrics, 97,* 424–436.

Price, C. (1989). Continuous renal replacement therapy, from a professional nursing perspective. *Nephrology News and Issues, 3*(7), 31–34.

Ragland, G. (1990). Electrolyte abnormalities in the alcoholic patient. *Emergency Medicine Clinics of North America, 8*(4), 761–771.

Robson, A. (1997). Parenteral fluid therapy. In R. Behrman (Ed.), *Nelson textbook of pediatrics* (14th ed., pp. 171–211). Philadelphia: Saunders.

Rose, B. D. (1997). *Clinical physiology of acid-base and electrolyte disorders* (3rd ed.). New York: McGraw-Hill.

Ross Roundtable Report, 12th. (1992). Enteral nutrition support for the 1990's: Innovations in nutrition, technology and techniques. Columbus, OH: Ross Laboratories (Division of Abbott Laboratories).

Rutherford, C. (1989). Fluid and electrolyte therapy: Considerations for patient care. *Journal of Intravenous Nursing, 12*(3), 175–183.

Salem, M., Munoz, R., & Chernow, B. (1991). Hypomagnesemia in critical illness. *Critical Care Clinics, 7*(1), 225–247.

Samson, L. F., & Ouzts, K. M. (1996). Fluid and electrolyte regulation. In M. Curley, J. Smith, & P. Moloney-Harmon (Eds.), *Critical care nursing of infants and children* (pp. 385–409). Philadelphia: Saunders.

Schrier, R. W. (1997). *Renal and electrolyte disorders* (3rd ed.). Boston: Little, Brown.

Shakir, K. M. M., & Amin, R. M. (1991). Hypoglycemia. *Critical Care Clinics, 7*(1), 75–87.

Smith, Z. H., & VanGeilick, A. J. (1992). Management of neutropenic enterocolitis in the patient with cancer. *Oncology Nursing Forum, 19,* 1337–1342.

Sommers, M. (1990). Rapid fluid resuscitation: How to correct dangerous deficits. *Nursing 1990, 20*(1), 52–60.

Stein, J. H. (1988, March 30). Hypokalemia: Common and uncommon causes. *Hospital Practice.*

Sterns, R. H. (1991). The management of hyponatremic emergencies. *Critical Care Clinics, 7*(1), 127–141.

Szerlip, H., & Goldfarb, S. (1993). *Fluid and electrolyte disorders.* New York: Churchill Livingstone.

Terry, J. (1994). The major electrolytes. *Journal of Intravenous Nursing, 17*(5), 240–247.

Twombly, M. (1983). Shift to third space. *Monitoring fluid and electrolytes precisely: Nursing skillbook.* Horsham, PA: Intermed Communications.

Valle, G. A., & Lemberg, L. (1988). Electrolyte imbalances in cardiovascular disease: The forgotten factor. *Heart and Lung, 17*(3), 324–329.

VanHook, J. W. (1991). Hypermagnesemia. *Critical Care Clinics, 7*(1), 215–223.

Votey, S. R., Peters, A. L., & Hoffman, J. R. (1989). Disorders of water metabolism: Hyponatremia and hypernatremia. *Emergency Medicine Clinics of North America, 7*(4), 749–765.

Watkins, S. L. (1995). The basics of fluid and electrolyte therapy. *Pediatric Annuals, 24*(1), 16–22.

Watson, J. E. (1987). Fluid and electrolyte disorders in cardiovascular patients. *Nursing Clinics of North America, 22*(4), 797–803.

Wittaker, A. (1985). Acute renal dysfunction. *Focus on Critical Care, 12*(3), 12–17.

Wong, D. (1998). *Essentials of pediatric nursing* (4th ed.). Philadelphia: Mosby-Year Book.

Wong, D. L. (1999). *Whaley & Wong's nursing care of infants and children* (6th ed.). St. Louis: Mosby.

Young, M. E., & Flynn, K. T. (1988). Third-spacing. When the body conceals fluid loss. *RN, 51*(8), 46–48.

Zalaga, G. P. (1991). Hypocalcemic crisis. *Critical Care Clinics, 7*(1), 191–199.

Zull, D. N. (1989). Disorders of potassium metabolism. *Emergency Medicine Clinics of North America, 7*(1), 771–793.

Index

('b' indicates boxed material, 'i' indicates an illustration, 't' indicates a table)